S fu wou

MCQs for Dentistry

Second Edition

Kathleen FM Fan PhD, MBBS, BDS, FDSRCS (Eng), FRCS (Ed), FRCS (OMFS)
Consultant Oral and Maxillofacial Surgeon
King's College Hospital, London / Queen Mary's Hospital, Sidcup

Judith Jones BDS, MSc, FDSRCS (Eng), PhD, FDS (OS), FHEA
Senior Clinical Lecturer / Honorary Consultant
Department of Oral Surgery, Queen Mary University of London,
Barts and The London School of Medicine and Dentistry, Institute of Dentistry

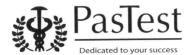

PasTest
Dedicated to your success

© 2010 PASTEST LTD
Egerton Court
Parkgate Estate
Knutsford
Cheshire
WA16 8DX

Telephone: 01565 752000

First Published 2006
Second Edition Published 2010

ISBN: 1905635575
         9781905635573

A catalogue record for this book is available from the British Library.

The information contained within this book was obtained by the authors from reliable sources. However, while every effort has been made to ensure its accuracy, no responsibility for loss, damage or injury occasioned to any person acting or refraining from action as a result of information contained herein can be accepted by the publishers or authors.

PasTest Revision Books and Intensive Courses

PasTest has been established in the field of undergraduate and postgraduate medi-cal education since 1972, providing revision books and intensive study courses for doctors preparing for their professional examinations.

Books and courses are available for:
Medical undergraduates, MRCGP, MRCP Parts 1 and 2, MRCPCH Parts 1 and 2, MRCS, MRCOG Parts 1 and 2, DRCOG, DCH, FRCA, Dentistry.

For further details contact:
PasTest, Freepost, Knutsford, Cheshire WA16 7BR
Tel: 01565 752000   **Fax: 01565 650264**
www.pastest.co.uk   **enquiries@pastest.co.uk**

Text prepared by Carnegie Publishing
Printed and bound in the UK by CPI Antony Rowe

Contents

Contributors

Julia Costello BDS MSc
Clinical Demonstrator, Department of Periodontology
Guy's Hospital, Kings College London

Mandeep Ghuman BDS BSc(Hons) MFDS RCS (Eng)
Senior House Officer
Kent & Canterbury Hospital
Canterbury, Kent

Introduction

Multiple choice questions have been used for many years as a way of testing a candidate's knowledge and recall of information. Over the years, they have been in and out of vogue but a lot of courses have seen a resurgence in their usage recently. The cynics amongst you may think that MCQs are popular because they are easy to mark. Whatever the reason, they are an accepted and frequently used method of testing knowledge.

The MCQs in this book are of the "true/false" variety. The questions will start with a statement or stem followed by a group of phrases. You need to mark each statement as to whether you think it is true or false. Each phrase is independent of the others in the group and there can be any combination of true and false phrases in a question.

The aim is to get as many marks as possible so it is necessary to know how the questions are going to be marked. For example, if negative marking is used then you receive a mark for each correct answer and have a mark deducted for each wrong answer. This is important to know as guessing in this type of test will cause you to lose marks. However, if there is no negative marking it is possible to guess answers without losing marks.

When doing MCQs, it is important to read the questions carefully and read what is written and not what you expect to read. For example, there are often little things in them to trip you up like double negatives. Rest assured, we have tried not to incorporate them in the questions in this book. Another tip is to look for questions that include words like "always" and "never" as these are often false. Each question usually has the same amount of marks so it is important to do the whole paper.

As with most things, the only way to get good at MCQs is to practise them and this book will provide you with an opportunity to do that. Each question has the true answers listed on the following page and a short explanation about the questions to help your revision.

This book is intended to help you practise MCQs to prepare for examinations in dentistry and is suitable for both undergraduates and postgraduates students. We hope you find it useful and wish you every success in your forthcoming examinations.

Judith Jones & Kathy Fan

1

General
Dentistry

1.1 **Which of the following statements regarding oral hygiene methods and adjuncts are correct?**

A   The Bass tooth brushing technique is a sulcular technique in which the bristles of the brush are directed into the sulcus at a 45° angle to the long axis of the tooth and the brush is rolled to sweep the bristles over the tooth and gingivae

B   The Bass tooth brushing technique is particularly good for disrupting the plaque biofilm and for cleaning under the gingival margin provided that no pockets are greater than 3 mm in depth

C   The Charter tooth brushing technique is particularly good after periodontal surgery and for patients wearing orthodontic appliances

D   The Fones circular technique is particularly good to use when patients are not exceptionally manually dexterous, eg children

E   Natural bristle toothbrushes are no longer used as the bristles are often of differing lengths, thicknesses and durability, even though they are more hygienic than nylon ones

1.2 **Which of the following statements are true regarding sterilisers that are commonly used in the dental environment?**

A   Type B sterilisers incorporate a vacuum stage and so can be used for packaged and hollow instruments

B   Type B sterilisers are non-vacuum sterilisers and are unsuitable for packaged or hollow instruments

C   Type N sterilisers incorporate a vacuum stage and so can be used for packaged and hollow instruments

D   Type N sterilisers are non-vacuum sterilisers and are unsuitable for packaged or hollow instruments

E   Type S sterilisers are designed to process specific load types and hence should only be used for the appropriate load

1.1 BCD

In the Bass technique the brush is directed into the sulcus at a 45° angle to the long axis of the tooth and the brush is moved backwards and forwards in short strokes. In the Charter technique the bristle tips are directed towards the occlusal surface at a 45° angle to the long axis of the tooth and the brush is moved backwards and forwards. Hence this technique is good for patients wearing fixed orthodontic appliances and in the immediate wound healing phase after gingival surgery.

Natural bristle toothbrushes are no longer used for many reasons including the fact that the bristles are often of differing lengths, thicknesses and durability, but more importantly they are much more likely to harbour bacteria than nylon bristles as natural bristles are often hollow.

1.2 AD

The air removal in a type N steriliser occurs by passive displacement and so they should not be used for wrapped, hollow or air-retentive instruments. Type B on the other hand have a vacuum stage and so can be used for these instruments. Type S sterilisers are designed to process specific load types and hence should only be used for the appropriate load, which will be defined by the manufacturer.

1.3 **Which of the following information points should be contained in an infection control policy for dental practices?**

A   A policy for hand hygiene

B   A policy for disposal of clinical waste from high-risk patients

C   A policy for disposal of patient records and radiographs

D   A policy for the use of personal protective equipment

E   A policy for decontamination of new reusable instruments

1.4 **The current principal methods of cleaning reusable dental instruments prior to sterilisation are:**

A   Autoclaving

B   Hot air oven

C   Manual cleaning

D   Manual cleaning and ultrasonic bath combined

E   Use of a washer-disinfector

1.3 ADE

All dental practices must have written infection control policies that contain information relating to all aspects of infection control. A policy for disposal of clinical waste forms part of this but there is no need to have a separate policy for disposal of waste from high-risk patients as universal precautions are used for all patients, and all patients should be treated equally with regard to infection control. There should be a practice policy on disposal of patient records but this is not related to infection control.

1.4 CDE

Instruments should be cleaned prior to sterilisation as this reduces the risk of transmission of infectious agents. Wherever possible, instruments should be cleaned using an automated washer-disinfector, because this includes a disinfection stage that renders the instruments safe for handling. Autoclaving and hot air ovens, although capable of sterilising instruments, do not clean them. More information is available in the Department of Health publication *Health Technical Memorandum 01–05* (October 2008).

1.5   Which of the following are principles of good hand hygiene?

A   Liquid soap should be applied to the hands prior to water to get maximum benefit from the soap

B   Effective drying of hands is not necessary after hand washing

C   Hand hygiene is not required during decontamination of instruments as gloves are used, hence preventing any microbes on the skin surface reaching the instruments and vice versa

D   Liquid soap or bar soap may be used in a dental practice setting for hand hygiene

E   If an antibacterial solution is used to clean the hands prior to donning non-sterile gloves for clinical work it is not necessary to remove rings and bracelets as the solution will minimise the numbers of bacteria on jewellery and skin

1.6   Which of the following are correct definitions of terms commonly used in healthcare?

A   The prevalence of a disease is the number of cases in a given population at a specific time point

B   The incidence of a disease is the number of cases in a given population at a specific time point

C   The prevalence of a disease is the number of new cases in a given population appearing over a specific period of time

D   The incidence of a disease is the number of new cases in a given population appearing over a specific period of time

E   Primary prevention aims to arrest disease through early detection and treatment

1.5   All statements are false

- Soap should be applied to wet hands to minimise the risk of irritation and handwashing should be performed under running water.
- Hands should be dried after washing as wet surfaces transfer microorganisms more easily; plus there is a greater risk of skin damage if hands are not dried.
- Bar soap has the potential to harbour microbes and hence liquid soap is preferable.
- Hand hygiene is required for decontamination of dental instruments, as wearing of gloves is not a substitute for good hand hygiene.
- Ideally, all jewellery would be removed prior to cleaning hands with any hand cleaning material for clinical work. However, because of social reasons it is acceptable for a plain wedding band to be left on. This does, however, increase the risk of skin irritation under the ring so special care should be taken to ensure the skin is washed and thoroughly dried.

1.6   AD

Secondary prevention aims to arrest disease through early detection and treatment. Primary prevention seeks to prevent the initial occurrence of a disease or disorder and so targets healthy individuals.

1.7 **At which of the following autoclave conditions would sterilisation be achieved?**

A   121 °C for 15 minutes

B   121 °C for 5 minutes

C   121 °C for 3 minutes

D   134 °C for 3 minutes

E   134 °C for 5 minutes

1.8 **Which of the following requirements must be satisfied when gaining informed consent from a patient?**

A   The patient has a chaperone

B   The consent is voluntary

C   A written list of warnings must be given to the patient

D   The patient understands the treatment plan

E   The patient is over 18 years of age

1.9 **Which of the following are responsibilities of the General Dental Council?**

A   Registration of dentists

B   Registration of dental practices

C   Protection of the public

D   Professional indemnity

E   Ensuring continuing professional development

1.7 ADE

Recommended autoclave cycles are usually 121 °C for 15 minutes or 134 °C for 3 minutes. Sterilisation will also be achieved at 134 °C for 5 minutes but is not necessary as it is already achieved at 3 minutes at this temperature.

1.8 BD

Consent can only be gained when the procedure, the consequences of not carrying out the procedure and alternative treatments have been explained to the patient. All the risks, complications and benefits of the procedure must be explained, and the patient should understand the information given. Consent must be voluntary. Patients under 16 years of age may give consent for treatment provided they understand the above conditions (Gillick competence).

1.9 ACE

The General Dental Council is the regulatory body of the dental profession. It protects the public by means of its statutory responsibility for registration, dental education and professional conduct and health. It also supports dentists in the practice of dentistry and encourages their continuing professional development.

1.10 **Which of the following protocols must be included in the 'written practice protocols'?**

  A Disposal of hazardous waste

  B Disposal of sharps

  C Annual leave entitlements

  D Radiation protection

  E Autoclaving

1.11 **Who may be given access to a patient's dental records without their permission?**

  A The patient's spouse/partner

  B The patient's employer

  C An insurance/defence organisation if it is investigating an allegation of negligence

  D A court of law

  E The patient's parents

1.12 **Which of the following conditions must be met in order to prove dental negligence?**

  A The patient was not happy with the treatment as it was of a poor standard

  B The dentist had a duty of care to the patient

  C The patient was overcharged for the treatment

  D Duty of care was breached

  E Breach of care resulted in damage

1.10 ABDE

Written practice protocols should include information on radiation protection, cleaning and sterilization of instruments and impressions, disposal of sharps and hazardous waste, protective clothing and medical history forms.

1.11 CD

Confidentiality is almost always absolute. However, there are a few circumstances when patient information may be passed on. For example, records may be passed to other healthcare professionals treating the patient or to an insurance company/defence organisation in relation to a claim. Occasionally there may be a legal requirement, for example to disclose information to a court of law or if there is a notifiable infectious disease. In addition, dental records may have to be released for the purpose of identifying missing persons.

1.12 BDE

In order for a claimant (or patient) to prove that a dentist was negligent they must prove that the dentist had a duty of care which was breached and that this resulted in harm or injury.

1.13 Which of the following statements about fluoride are true?

A Fluoride has an effect on enamel only if it is given while the tooth is forming

B Fluoride is absorbed mainly from the duodenum and is excreted by the kidneys

C Fluoride is absorbed mainly from the stomach and is excreted by the kidneys

D Fluoride is more effective at decreasing pit and fissure caries than smooth surface caries

E Fluoride is more effective at decreasing smooth surface caries than pit and fissure caries

1.14 Which of the following cross-infection control measures should be adopted by all dental personnel?

A Immunisation against hepatitis B

B Immunisation against hepatitis C

C Immunisation against hepatitis A

D Wearing of gloves when treating patients

E Wearing of eye protection

1.15 Which of the following are known to be risk factors for oral cancer?

A Tobacco consumption

B Social deprivation

C Alcohol consumption

D High levels of stress

E Previous trauma to the site

1.13   CE

Fluoride has an effect on enamel both while the tooth is forming and after eruption. It is absorbed from the stomach and excreted via the kidneys.

1.14   ADE

Universal cross-infection control measures should be taken when treating all patients. These include immunisation against hepatitis B and wearing gloves, masks and eye protection as well as protective clothing. At present there is no vaccination available against hepatitis C. Hepatitis A is a viral infection that is spread via the oro-faecal route, and is unlikely to be transmitted by dental treatment, especially where universal precautions are employed.

1.15   ABC

Risk factors for oral cancer include tobacco smoking, tobacco chewing, snuff usage, betel nut chewing, alcohol consumption and social deprivation. Previous trauma and stress are not thought to have an effect.

1.16 **Which of the following foodstuffs/drinks contain fluoride not added by the manufacturer/supplier?**

    A   Coffee

    B   Tea

    C   Salt

    D   Bony fish

    E   Wine

1.17 **Deposition of local anaesthetic solution close to the left lingula of the mandible is likely to anaesthetise the:**

    A   Left side of the anterior aspect of the tongue

    B   Labial gingivae on the left

    C   Buccal gingivae of the left lower molars

    D   Left side of the posterior third of the tongue

    E   Pulp of the lower molars on the left

1.18 **Clinical records for adults should be kept for:**

    A   3 years

    B   5 years

    C   7 years

    D   11 years

    E   15 years

1.16   BD

Bony fish, tea and beer contain naturally occurring fluoride.

1.17   ABE

Depositing local anaesthetic in the region of the left lingula will anaesthetise the left inferior dental nerve, and hence the pulps of the lower teeth and the labial gingivae on the left will go numb. As the lingual nerve lies close to the lingula it is also possible to anaethetise it, so the left side of the anterior aspect of the tongue will go numb. The posterior aspect of the tongue is supplied by the glossopharyngeal and vagus nerves. The long buccal nerve supplies the buccal gingivae of the lower molars.

1.18   D

All clinical records should be kept for 11 years for adults. For children, clinical records should be kept until the individual is 25 years old or for 11 years, whichever is longer.

1.19 **If a person has undergone a course of vaccination against the hepatitis B virus, which of the following antibody levels would imply that they have responded to the vaccination and are protected against catching the infection?**

A   HbsAb > 1 mIU/ml

B   HbsAb > 10 mIU/ml

C   HbsAb > 100 mIU/ml

D   HbsAg > 1000 mIU/ml

E   None of the above

1.20 **Which of the following are essential features of cariogenic bacteria:**

A   Ability to attach to the smooth surface of a tooth

B   Ability to produce acid with an appropriate pH (pH > 6) to decalcify tooth substance

C   Ability to survive in stagnant areas

D   Ability to form insoluble glucans

E   Ability to metabolise sugar alcohols (polyols)

1.21 **Dental hygienists are allowed to:**

A   Record periodontal probing depths

B   Record mobility of teeth

C   Give oral hygiene instruction

D   Give inferior dental nerve blocks under supervision

E   Take dental impressions

1.19   CD

Protection against hepatitis B usually occurs with HbsAg antibody levels greater than 100 mIU/ml.

1.20   AD

The bacteria need to be able to produce enough acid so that the pH drops to < 5. The cariogenicity of *Streptococcus mutans* stems from its ability to produce large amounts of insoluble glucans (to enable adhesion) and acid. Sugar alcohols are non-cariogenic, eg sorbitol.

1.21   ABC

Hygienists may only work under the supervision of a registered dentist and the treatment plan must be written down and less than a year old. They are allowed to record probing depths and tooth mobility, and give oral hygiene instruction. They should not take impressions or give inferior dental nerve blocks, even under supervision.

1.22 **With respect to continuing professional development (CPD), a dentist must carry out:**

A   75 hours of CPD of which 25 must be certifiable over a year

B   150 hours of CPD of which 50 must be certifiable over a year

C   200 hours of CPD of which 75 must be certifiable over a 5-year period

D   250 hours of CPD of which 75 must be certifiable over a 5-year period

E   CPD is left up to the individual dentist's needs

1.23 **With regard to dental nomenclature systems:**

A   An upper right first permanent molar may be written as 26 using the World Dental Federation (FDI) system

B   An upper right first permanent molar may be written as 16 using the FDI system

C   A lower left deciduous canine may be written as 33 using the FDI system

D   A lower left deciduous canine may be written as 43 using the FDI system

E   A lower left deciduous canine may be written as 3C using the FDI system

1.24 **When disposing of waste from a dental practice, it is important to separate waste into the appropriate category for disposal (clinical, non-clinical and special waste). Which of the following are examples of special waste?**

A   Blood-stained gauze

B   Radiography fixer solution

C   Alginate impression

D   Half a cartridge of 2% lidocaine and 1:80 000 adrenaline (epinephrine)

E   Mercury

1.22   D

'CPD' means studying, training, attending courses and seminars, reading and other activities undertaken by a dentist, which could reasonably be expected to advance their professional development as a dentist. CPD is mandatory for all registered dentists. A 'CPD cycle' is a 5-year period and dentists must complete 250 hours of CPD of which 75 hours are verifiable. Dentists should keep up-to-date records of the CPD that they undertake and submit these to the General Dental Council on demand.

1.23   B

The quadrants are numbered as follows:

- Upper right permanent – 1
- Upper left permanent – 2
- Lower left permanent – 3
- Lower right permanent – 4
- Upper right deciduous – 5
- Upper left deciduous – 6
- Lower left deciduous – 7
- Lower right deciduous – 8

Permanent and deciduous teeth are numbered 1–8 and 1–5, respectively, in each quadrant starting from the midline. Hence the upper right first permanent molar would be written as 16 and the lower left deciduous canine would be written as 73.

1.24 BDE

All mercury waste and radiography developer and fixative solutions must be disposed of as special waste, as must all prescribed medicines. As local anaesthetic is in effect a prescribed medicine it is treated as special waste. Anything contaminated with body fluids should be disposed of in the clinical waste, eg impressions and blood-stained gauze.

2
Human
Disease

2.1   A patient presenting to your dental surgery requires extraction of a
      lower second premolar. In his medical history he states that he has a
      monthly international normalised ratio (INR) test, and previously had
      an INR prior to a dental extraction. However, he cannot remember the
      name of his medication. Which of the following medication would he
      have taken, which is monitored by an INR prior to dental extractions?

      A   Clopidogrel

      B   Enoxaparin

      C   Heparin

      D   Vitamin K

      E   Warfarin

2.2   Which of the following statements are true regarding the various
      types of diabetes mellitus?

      A   Type 2 is commonly caused by destruction of the pancreatic islet cells
          leading to insulin insufficiency

      B   Type 2 diabetes is often associated with obesity

      C   The onset of type 1 diabetes is usually in younger patients (less than 30
          years)

      D   Gestational diabetes is always controlled by diet alone

      E   Patients with type 1 diabetes are more likely to get ketosis than those
          with type 2 diabetes

2.1   E

- Clopidogrel is an anti-platelet drug that is used to prevent atherosclerotic events. Patients taking anti-platelet drugs are not monitored by an INR test prior to dental extractions.

- Heparin and enoxaparin, which is a low molecular weight heparin, inhibit clotting by neutralising the action of thrombin on fibrinogen and preventing the activation of prothrombin to thrombin. Patients on heparins tend to have a normal INR but their thrombin time will be increased, hence an INR is not used as a routine test for patients on these drugs.

- Vitamin K is required for the synthesis of prothrombin (factor II) and factors VII, IX and X in the liver. Lack of vitamin K will cause clotting time to be increased.

- Warfarin is an anti-coagulant that is monitored by regular INR tests, and patients having dental extractions must have an INR check no more than 72 hours prior to the extraction. For more information, see the National Patient Safety Agency (NPSA) website (www.npsa.nhs.uk).

2.2   BCE

Type 1 diabetes mellitus usually has its onset in childhood but can affect any age; there is deficiency of insulin, which may be caused by the destruction of the pancreatic islet cells. Type 2 diabetes is often seen in older age groups and obese patients and is due to impaired insulin secretion or insulin resistance. Gestational diabetes may require medical management, not just diet control.

2.3 **Which of the following statements about the dental relevance of diabetes mellitus are correct?**

A   Patients must have antibiotics after dental extractions as they are more susceptible to infection

B   Timing of dental appointments is important and patients should be treated before mealtimes

C   Timing of dental appointments is important and patients should be treated after mealtimes

D   Only patients with type 1 diabetes are more prone to rapidly progressing periodontal disease

E   Patients with diabetes often have oral dysaesthesia (burning mouth)

2.4 **For which of the following conditions might a patient be taking bisphosphonate drugs?**

A   Bone metastases from breast cancer

B   Multiple myeloma

C   Odontogenic myxoma

D   Osteoporosis

E   Osteoradionecrosis

2.3   CE

Patients with diabetes are more susceptible to all kinds of infections but there is no blanket rule that patients having extractions must have antibiotics post extraction. Instead each patient is treated individually and antibiotics prescribed if indicated. Patients with either type 1 or type 2 diabetes are more prone to periodontal disease than patients without diabetes. Timing of appointments is important so as not to interrupt normal eating and drug taking patterns, hence it is ideal is to see patient as soon as possible after a meal so that all treatment is finished before the patient can become hypoglycaemic. People with diabetes are also more prone to oral dysaesthesia than non-diabetic patients.

2.4   ABD

Bisphosphonates are inhibitors of osteoclast function and are used for prevention and treatment of certain bone disorders. In particular they are used to prevent and treat osteoporosis, and to treat Paget's disease, osteogenesis imperfecta and metastatic bone disease (often in connection with breast or prostrate cancer) and multiple myeloma. Osteoradionecrosis is not treated with bisphosphonates. Odontogenic myxomas are benign tumours of the dental mesenchymal tissues which are treated by excision.

2.5 **Which of the following statements regarding asthmatic patients are correct?**

A   Patients with asthma should not be given non-steroidal anti-inflammatory drugs (NSAIDs), as this may precipitate an asthma attack

B   Patients with asthma should not be given codeine-based analgesic drugs as they may precipitate an asthma attack

C   Patients with asthma should not be given intravenous sedation in a practice setting

D   Asthmatic patients should rinse their mouth out after using salbutamol inhalers as this will reduce the risk of them getting oral candidiasis

E   Patients with severe asthma should not be given local anaesthetic that contains adrenaline (epinephrine) as a vasoconstrictor as this may precipitate an asthma attack

2.6 **Which of the following statements regarding serological markers of viral hepatitis are correct?**

A   Presence of the HBsAg (the surface antigen) alone implies that the patient had a previous infection but is low risk with regard to transmitting the infection

B   Presence of the HBsAg (the surface antigen) alone implies that the patient had a previous infection but is high risk with regard to transmitting the infection

C   The HBcAg (the core antigen) if present in serum means that the patient is highly infective

D   The HBeAg (the hepatitis E antigen) if present in serum means that the patient is highly infective

E   The antibody to HBsAg will only be present if the patient has been successfully immunised against HBsAg

2.5   All statements are false

It is thought that only about 10% of asthmatic people have a reaction when given NSAIDs, hence it is sensible to ask patients if they have ever taken any NSAID drugs before and if they have had a reaction to them prior to prescribing analgesics. Codeine-based drugs do not precipitate asthma attacks. The decision on whether to administer intravenous sedation to any patient with respiratory disease will depend on the severity of the disease. People with mild asthma can safely be treated with sedation in a practice setting, but those with more severe disease will require specialist treatment.

In order to minimise the risk of oropharyngeal candidal infections it is advisable to rinse the mouth out after using steroid-based inhalers, but not β_2-agonist based inhalers such as salbutamol. Adrenaline (epinephrine) has both α- and β-adrenergic properties hence helps with bronchodilation, so local anaesthetic with adrenaline (epinephrine) as a vasoconstrictor is safe to use in asthmatic patients.

2.6   AD

Presence of HBsAg implies that the patient had a previous infection but is low risk with regard to transmitting the infection unless HBeAg is also present. HBcAg is only present in the liver, not in serum. HBeAg appears in the serum at the same time as HBsAg when a patient is infected but HBeAg disappears when there is full recovery. If HBeAg persists it implies that the patient is highly infective. Antibodies to HBsAg can be present following successful immunisation to hepatitis B or they can be present if the patient mounted their own immune response to infection with hepatitis B.

2.7 **Which of the following conditions might make a patient susceptible to infective endocarditis following dental treatment?**

A   Previous history of rheumatic fever

B   Presence of a cardiac pacemaker

C   Congenital cardiac lesion

D   Diagnosis of atrial fibrillation

E   Heart murmur

2.8 **A patient tells you that they have had hepatitis. Which of the following may be of concern when providing dental treatment for them?**

A   The patient will need antibiotic cover for invasive procedures

B   Increased bleeding following invasive procedures due to impaired synthesis of clotting factors

C   High risk of infective endocarditis after extractions

D   Possible cross-infection risk

E   Impaired drug metabolism

2.7 ACE

Patients who have valvular defects, either congenital in origin or developing after rheumatic fever, patients with congenital cardiac defects, and patients with aortic regurgitation, mitral regurgitation and aortic stenosis are at risk of infective endocarditis following bacteraemia. However, according to the National Institute for Health and Clinical Excellence (NICE) guidelines published in 2008 antibiotic prophylaxis is no longer required for any dental treatment (see www.nice.org.uk).

However, NICE does recommend that patients at risk of infective endocarditis should be offered information about prevention, including the risks and benefits of antibiotic cover, an explanation of why antibiotic prophylaxis is no longer routinely recommended as well as the importance of maintaining good oral health and symptoms that may indicate infective endocarditis and when to seek expert advice.

Patient with cardiac pacemakers or atrial fibrillation are not at an increased risk of infective endocarditis.

2.8   BDE

Patients with liver disease are likely to have disordered clotting and abnormal drug metabolism. If their disease is due to infective hepatitis there may be a risk of cross-infection. Prophylactic antibiotic cover is not required for patients with liver disease, nor are they susceptible to infective endocarditis following extractions.

See Answer 2.7 regarding antibiotic prophylaxis.

2.9 **Which of the following statements about Down's syndrome are true?**

 A   It is caused by trisomy 20

 B   It is caused by trisomy 21

 C   The incidence increases with increasing age of the mother

 D   Patients with Down's syndrome often have delayed eruption of teeth

 E   Patients with Down's syndrome often have microglossia

 F   Patients with Down's syndrome often have congenital cardiac defects

2.10 **Which of the following statements regarding the Resuscitation Council's (UK) recommendations of the ratio of compressions to breaths per minute are/is correct?**

 A   Depends on the number of rescuers

 B   Use a ratio of 30 compressions to 2 rescue breaths if there are two rescuers

 C   Use a ratio of 15 compressions to 2 rescue breaths if there is one rescuer

 D   Use a ratio of 5 compressions to 1 rescue breath if there are two rescuers

 E   Use a ratio of 5 compressions to 1 rescue breath if there is one rescuer

2.11 **Which of the following are recommended by the Resuscitation Council (UK) when performing basic life support on an adult?**

 A   Ensure safety of rescuer and victim

 B   If victim is not breathing, give two slow, effective rescue breaths and then go for help if you are alone

 C   Look, listen and feel for 20 seconds to determine if the victim is breathing normally

 D   Assess the victim for signs of circulation by checking the radial pulse

 E   If there are no signs of circulation, start external cardiac compression by applying pressure over the left side of the chest

2.9   BCDF

Down's syndrome is a condition caused by trisomy 21. Its incidence increases with increasing age of the mother. Patients often have delayed eruption of teeth, macroglossia and congenital cardiac lesions.

2.10   B

Current Resuscitation Council (UK) guidelines advise using the same ratio for both one and two rescuers. The aim is 100 compressions per minute, and 30 compressions to 2 rescue breaths. New guidelines were published at the end of 2005, with changed compression : breath ratio (see www.resus.org.uk).

2.11   A

The first priority is safety and so the rescuer should be aware of any potential risks associated with attempting to resuscitate a victim and these risks should be eliminated or minimised prior to attempting resuscitation. If the victim is not breathing or is only making occasional gasps or weak attempts at breathing, send someone for help. If you are on your own, leave the victim and go for assistance.

Assess the circulation by looking, listening and feeling for normal breathing, coughing or movement by the victim, and check the carotid pulse within 10 seconds if trained to do so. The radial pulse is not used to assess the circulation in this situation. External cardiac compression is performed by pressing over the middle of victim's chest and not on the left side.

2.12 **A patient complains of severe chest pain while in your dental chair. Appropriate management includes:**

    A   Lie the patient flat

    B   Lie the patient in the recovery position

    C   Administer sublingual glyceryl trinitrate (GTN)

    D   Give the patient oxygen

    E   Administer Hypostop® gel buccally

2.13 **You have a patient with known diabetes who becomes sweaty in the dental chair. How would you manage this situation?**

    A   Continue with what you are doing and aim to finish quickly

    B   Check if the patient had eaten and give them some glucose

    C   Check if the patient had eaten and give them some insulin

    D   Check their blood glucose (BM)

    E   Try to calm the patient as they are probably anxious

2.14 **Anaphylaxis:**

    A   Is caused by an acute-type intravenous allergic response

    B   Results in acute hypertension, bronchospasm and urticaria

    C   Is managed by laying the patient flat and maintaining the airway

    D   Is managed by giving 0.5 ml of 1:1000 adrenaline (epinephrine) intravenously

    E   Is managed by giving oxygen

2.12   CD

Lying the patient flat may make their breathing more difficult, so this is not advised. Sublingual GTN can be given as the pain may be due to angina. Hypostop® gel is a glucose-containing gel that is used in hypoglycaemic events.

2.13   BD

Diabetic patients could forget to eat prior to their appointment and may be hypoglycaemic. If there is doubt whether the patient has hypo/hyperglycaemia it is safer to give the patient glucose as it will do no immediate harm to the hyperglycaemic patient but may save the hypoglycaemic patient.

If there are signs that the patient is not well, it is always best to abort the procedure and deal with the medical issues.

2.14   CE

Anaphylaxis is caused by a type I hypersensitivity reaction during which histamine is released from mast cells. This causes acute hypotension, bronchospasm and urticaria. Management involves laying the patient flat, maintaining the airway and giving drugs including 0.5 ml of 1:1000 adrenaline (epinephrine) intramuscularly and oxygen.

2.15 With regard to the following emergencies, which commonly used drugs and doses are correct?

A Anaphylaxis – 0.5 ml of 1:100 adrenaline (epinephrine) solution intramuscularly

B Anaphylaxis – 10–20 mg chlorphenamine intravenously

C Diabetic collapse – 20 units of insulin subcutaneously

D Steroid collapse – 100–200 mg hydrocortisone sodium succinate intravenously

E Diabetic collapse – 10 mg glucagon intramuscularly

2.16 The following sites are frequently used for intramuscular injections:

A Vastus lateralis

B Deltoid

C Gluteal muscle

D Antecubital fossa

E Dorsum of the hand

2.15 BD

In anaphylaxis, 0.5 ml of 1:1000 adrenaline (epinephrine) solution is given intramuscularly and 10–20 mg intravenous chlorphenamine is also used. In a diabetic collapse, insulin should never be given in an emergency situation. It is only used when the blood glucose level is known. Glucagon 1 mg intramuscularly can be given.

2.16 ABC

There are eight possible sites where intramuscular injections can be given, four on either side of the body: vastus lateralis muscle (thigh), deltoid muscle (upper arm), and ventrogluteal and dorsal gluteal muscles.

2.17 **Pregnant women:**

A   Can present with an epulis

B   Rarely get gingivitis

C   May become hypotensive when supine

D   Can take aspirin safely

E   Must always be given prilocaine (Citanest) and felypressin as a local anaesthetic

2.18 **Patients with which of the following conditions/drug treatment regimens may be at risk of an addisonian crisis?**

A   Addison's disease

B   Diabetes insipidus

C   Secondary hypoadrenalism

D   Long-term steroid therapy

E   Cushing's disease

2.19 **Diabetic patients:**

A   Have reduced resistance to dental infection

B   Have faster healing following surgery

C   May have accelerated periodontal disease

D   Are more prone to dental cysts

E   Should not be given lidocaine and adrenaline (epinephrine) as a local anaesthetic

2.17 AC

In late pregnancy, some patients become hypotensive when supine as the pregnant uterus impedes venous return. Pregnant ladies often get gingivitis. Aspirin is best avoided in pregnancy as it can delay onset and increase duration of labour and increase blood loss, as well as causing premature closure of the fetal ductus arteriosus. Pregnant women can be given lidocaine and adrenaline (epinephrine) perfectly safely.

2.18 ACD

Addisonian crisis is likely to present either in patients on long-term steroids or in those with Addison's disease (primary hypoadrenalism) or secondary aldosteronism. The hypothalamic–pituitary–adrenal axis is suppressed or completely atrophies and cannot respond to additional demand. Adrenal insufficiency has an insidious presentation but may present as an emergency (addisonian crisis) with vomiting, abdominal pain, profound weakness and hypovolaemic shock.

Diabetes insipidus occurs due to either impaired vasopressin secretion or resistance to its action. This leads to polyuria, nocturia and polydipsia. Cushing's disease is characterised by excess glucocorticoid secretion resulting from inappropriate adrenocorticotropic hormone (ACTH) secretion from the pituitary.

2.19 AC

Diabetic patients have reduced resistance to infections and hence are more prone to periodontal disease. They have a slower rate of healing. They are not more prone to dental cysts and can be given lidocaine and adrenaline (epinephrine) safely.

2.20   **Which of the following measures are appropriate for managing a patient experiencing an addisonian crisis?**

   A   Place the patient in a horizontal position

   B   Give glucagon

   C   Give intravenous hydrocortisone

   D   Set up intravenous infusion of fluid

   E   Call for medical assistance

2.21   **Hb 9.5 g/dL, WBC 5.3 x 10^9/l, platelets 200 x 10^9/l, RBC 4.7 x 10^9/l, MCV 76 fl, MCH 21.8 pg. This blood film:**

   A   Is consistent with anaemia

   B   Shows microcytic anaemia

   C   Shows macrocytic anaemia

   D   Is consistent with iron deficiency anaemia

   E   Is consistent with vitamin B_{12} deficiency anaemia

2.22   **Features of Paget's disease include:**

   A   Hypercementosis of teeth, which causes difficulties when extractions are needed

   B   Alveolar ridges may increase in size, so that new dentures need to be made

   C   Radiographs of bone may show radiolucent areas along with sclerotic areas

   D   Patients may suffer from symptoms of compression of cranial nerves

   E   Development of osteosarcoma is a common consequence of Paget's disease

2.20 ACDE

Glucagon is given to diabetic patients experiencing hypoglycaemia. Placing the patient supine helps management of shock but watch out if the patient is vomiting.

2.21 ABD

Normal range of values

- Haemoglobin: 8.1–11.2 g/dL [mmol/l] (13.5–18.0 g/dL) (male); 7.4–9.9 g/dL [mmol/l] (11.5–16.0 g/dL) (female)
- WBC: $4-11 \times 10^9/l$
- Platelets: $150-400 \times 10^9/l$
- RBC: $3.8-4.8 \times 10^{12}/l$
- MCV: 80–100 fl (femtolitres)
- MCH: 27–32 pg (picograms)

Anaemia is decreased level of haemoglobin (Hb) in the blood. The features of various types of anaemia are shown in the table below.

	Type of anaemia		
	Microcytic, hypochromic	Normocytic/ normochromic	Macrocytic
Blood film findings	Low MCV; low MCH	Normal MCV and MCH	High MCV
Causes	Iron deficiency Thalassaemia Sideroblastic anaemia	Acute blood loss Anaemia of chronic disease	Vitamin B_{12} deficiency Folate deficiency

2.22 ABCD

Paget's disease is characterised by excessive osteoclastic bone resorption followed by disordered osteoblastic activity, leading to abundant new bone formation which is structurally weak and abnormal. Radiographs reveal radiolucencies and sclerotic areas, and there is also hypercementosis. Bone deposition may lead to compression of the cranial nerves as well as changes in the size and shape of the alveolar ridges. Osteogenic sarcoma is a complication, but it is rare.

2.23 **Patients with which of the following conditions may be on long-term anticoagulants?**

A   Atrial fibrillation

B   Previous deep vein thrombosis

C   Cardiac pacemakers

D   Prosthetic heart valves

E   Ventricular fibrillation

2.24 **Which of the following is recommended by the Resuscitation Council (UK)?**

A   A ratio of 5 breaths to 1 compression when a single person is carrying out basic life support (BLS)

B   A ratio of 5 breaths to 1 compression when two people are carrying out BLS

C   A ratio of 15 breaths to 2 compressions when a single person is carrying out BLS

D   A ratio of 15 breaths to 2 compressions when two people are carrying out BLS

E   A ratio of 30 breaths to 1 compression at all times

2.25 **A patient starts fitting in your dental chair. Appropriate management options include:**

A   Call for the emergency services immediately

B   Protect the patient from harm

C   Place a bite prop in the mouth to prevent the patient from biting the tongue

D   Give 0.5 ml of 1:1000 solution of adrenaline (epinephrine) intramuscularly

E   If the fitting does not stop after 5 minutes give 10–20 mg diazepam

2.26 **A patient who weighs 60 kg and is 1 m 50 cm in height would have the following body mass index (BMI):**

A   20

B   24

C   28

D   32

E   36

2.23 ABD

Patients with atrial fibrillation, prosthetic heart valves and a history of deep vein thrombosis are treated with long-term anticoagulants. Patients with cardiac pacemakers are not given anticoagulants. Ventricular fibrillation is not compatible with life – it is a condition that results in no cardiac output and occurs in a cardiac arrest situation.

2.24   All statements are false

The Resuscitation Council (UK) recommends 30 compressions to 2 breaths for BLS whether one or two people are carrying it out.

2.25 BE

Most fits can be managed in the dental surgery without calling the emergency services. If the fitting does not stop then assistance should be sought, and diazepam, if available, should be given. It is important to prevent the patient from hurting themselves, which would mean moving loose equipment out of the way. Do not try to put anything in the patient's mouth as they may bite you. Adrenaline (epinephrine) is not indicated – it is used in anaphylaxis.

2.26 B

BMI is weight (in kg) divided by height (in m^2). Hence this patient would have a BMI of 24.

2.27   The patient in Q 2.26 would be classified as:

   A   Underweight

   B   Normal

   C   Overweight

   D   Obese

   E   Severely obese

2.28   Anaemia:

   A   Is defined as haemoglobin level below 11.5 g/dl in females and
       13.5 g/dl in males

   B   Due to iron deficiency is usually macrocytic

   C   Due to folate deficiency is usually microcytic

   D   Can be easily assessed by looking at a patient's skin colour

   E   May occur in sickle cell disease

2.29   Which of the following are fat-soluble vitamins?

   A   Vitamin B_1

   B   Vitamin A

   C   Vitamin C

   D   Vitamin E

   E   Vitamin D

2.27 B

The different categories of BMI are shown in the table below

BMI	Description
<20	Underweight
20-25	Normal weight
25-30	Overweight
30-40	Obese
>40	Severely obese

Hence the patient in Q 2.26 would be described as having normal weight.

2.28 AE

Macrocytic anaemia is usually due to vitamin B_{12} or folate deficiency. Microcytic anaemia is usually due to iron deficiency. Skin pallor does not give a good indication of whether a person is anaemic or not. Conjunctival or mucosal pallor gives a better idea, although neither is an accurate way of measuring anaemia. Anaemia may occur in sickle cell disease.

2.29 BDE

Vitamins A, D and E are all fat soluble.

2.30 Regarding vitamin deficiency:

   A   Vitamin A deficiency causes scurvy

   B   Vitamin C deficiency causes beri beri

   C   Vitamin D deficiency results in skeletal decalcification

   D   Vitamin D deficiency in children causes rickets

   E   Vitamin D deficiency in children causes delayed tooth eruption

2.31 Which of the following are causes of finger clubbing?

   A   Bacterial endocarditis

   B   Bronchial carcinoma

   C   Congenital cyanotic cardiac disease

   D   Angina

   E   Chronic pulmonary suppuration

2.32 Features of bacterial endocarditis include:

   A   Boutonniére's deformity

   B   Night sweats

   C   History of recent dental extractions

   D   Splinter haemorrhages

   E   Finger clubbing

2.30 CDE

Vitamin C deficiency causes scurvy and vitamin A deficiency results in hyperkeratosis of the skin and visual problems. Beri beri is caused by thiamine (vitamin B_1) deficiency. Vitamin D deficiency causes skeletal problems including decalcification, which in children results in rickets and delayed tooth eruption.

2.31 ABCE

Finger clubbing is the term used to describe fingers where the nail is curved and there is a loss of the angle between the nail and the bed. It occurs in a variety of conditions including: cyanotic cardiac disease; bacterial endocarditis; bronchial carcinoma; liver cirrhosis; ulcerative colitis; conditions with intrathoracic pus, (eg empyema, bronchiectasis); oesophageal ulcers; and Hodgkin's disease. It does not occur in angina.

2.32 BCDE

Infective endocarditis (subacute bacterial endocarditis) is an infection of the endocardium or valvular endothelium of the heart. Clinical features include:

- Infection – fever, night sweats, weight loss and anaemia, splenomegaly, clubbing
- Valve destruction – changing heart murmur leading to heart failure
- Embolic phenomena, eg stroke
- Immune complex deposition – splinter haemorrhages, Roth's spots, Osler's nodes

Boutonniére's deformity of the fingers is seen in rheumatoid arthritis.

2.33 **Causes of hypertension include:**

A Conn's syndrome

B Crohn's disease

C Phaeochromocytoma

D Chronic glomerulonephritis

E Unknown

2.34 **Which of the following are concerns in patients who have undergone a transplant?**

A Reduced resistance to infection

B Xerostomia

C Caries

D Susceptibility to osteoradionecrosis following tooth extraction

E Bleeding tendency

2.35 **With respect to bleeding disorders:**

A The prothrombin time is normal in patients with haemophilia

B The activated partial thromboplastin time is normal in haemophilia A

C Haemophilia A affects women more frequently than men

D Haemophilia A is due to factor IX deficiency

E Bleeding due to von Willebrand's disease may be treated with desmopressin and factor VIII concentrate

2.33 ACDE

In more than 90% of cases of hypertension the cause is unknown. This is referred to as 'essential hypertension'. Secondary hypertension may be due to: renal disease; endocrine disease including Cushing's syndrome, phaeochromocytoma and acromegaly; coarctation of the aorta; pre-eclampsia; and drugs. Conn's syndrome is primary hyperaldosteronism, which causes hypokalaemia and hypernatraemia with hypertension.

2.34 AE

Patients on immunosuppressive drugs are more prone to infections. Bleeding tendencies can occur in renal transplant patients and those with deranged liver function.

2.35 AE

The activated partial thromboplastin time is increased in haemophilia A. Haemophilia A is inherited as an X-linked recessive disease. It affects 1:5000 males and is the result of factor VIII deficiency.

2.36 **Risk factors for ischaemic heart disease that may be modified by the patient include:**

A   Smoking

B   Hypotension

C   Lack of exercise

D   Hypercholesterolaemia

E   Gender

2.37 **Patients with Down's syndrome have:**

A   Macroglossia

B   Periodontal disease

C   Mouth ulcers

D   Delayed tooth eruption

E   Large pulp chambers

2.38 **Which of the following put patients at greater risk of deep vein thrombosis (DVT)?**

A   Being overweight

B   Being on the oral contraceptive pill

C   Early mobilisation following surgery

D   Trauma to a vessel wall

E   Thrombophlebitis

2.36 ACD

Smoking, lack of exercise and hypercholesterolaemia are all risk factors for ischaemic heart disease that a patient could alter. Being male puts a patient at greater risk of ischaemic heart disease, but is not controlled by the patient. Hypertension, not hypotension, is a risk factor.

2.37 ABD

Other features seen in Down's syndrome include: anterior open bite, maxillary hypoplasia, hypodontia, scrotal tongue, and cheilitis. Large pulp chambers are seen in hypophosphataemia.

2.38 ABDE

Risk factors for DVT include being overweight, taking the oral contraceptive pill, thrombophlebitis and trauma to a vessel wall. Early mobilisation after surgery reduces the risk of DVT.

2.39 With respect to fractures:

A In a simple fracture there is no communication between the bone and the exterior

B In a greenstick fracture the bone bends without actual separation of the fragments

C In a comminuted fracture there is communication between the bone and the exterior

D A complicated fracture occurs at the site of a disease process

E In an impacted fracture the bone ends are driven together

2.40 Common causes of haemoptysis (blood in the sputum) are:

A Bronchial carcinoma

B Asthma

C Pulmonary tuberculosis

D Pneumonia

E Bronchiectasis

2.41 An asthma attack may be caused by:

A Exercise

B Stress

C Animal dander

D Paracetamol

E Cigarette smoke

2.39 ABE

A comminuted fracture is one in which there are multiple segments of bone. A complicated fracture is one involving a vital structure, eg a fractured angle of the mandible involving the inferior dental nerve. A pathological fracture occurs at a disease site.

2.40 ACDE

Haemoptysis occurs in pneumonia, tuberculosis, bronchiectasis, bronchial carcinoma and mitral stenosis. It is not a usual feature of asthma.

2.41 ABCE

Common precipitating factors of asthma attacks are exercise, stress, cold weather, fumes, animal dander, cigarette smoke, infections and some drugs, eg propranolol, non-steroidal anti-inflammatory drugs (NSAIDs). Paracetamol does not usually precipitate asthma attacks.

2.42 Regarding the thyroid gland:

A Thyroid hormones increase the metabolism of the body

B In Hashimoto's disease there is autoimmune destruction of the thyroid gland

C Graves' disease is a type of hypothyroidism

D Patients who are hypothyroid often have lethargy, cold intolerance and dry hair

E Patients who are hyperthyroid often have breathlessness, palpitations, increased pulse rate and constipation

2.43 Typical features of an anaphylactic attack include:

A Itching

B Paraesthesia

C Facial flushing

D Bronchodilation

E Hypertension

2.44 Regarding malignant disease:

A Hodgkin's disease is a type of leukaemia

B Acute leukaemia is a common childhood malignancy

C Patients with leukaemia often have intra-oral bleeding

D Patients with multiple myeloma often suffer from bone lesions and pain

E Oral squamous cell carcinomas are usually treated with chemotherapy

2.45 A patient gives a history of rheumatic fever. Which of the following procedures require prophylactic antibiotic cover?

A Scale and polish

B Extraction of a tooth

C Inferior dental nerve block

D Impression for a new lower complete denture

E Placing a class I amalgam restoration

2.42 ABD

Graves' disease is a type of hyperthyroidism. Hyperthyroid patients often have breathlessness, palpitations, increased pulse rate and frequent bowel movements.

2.43 ABC

The following signs and symptoms may occur during anaphylactic attacks: facial flushing, itching and paraesthesia, facial oedema, bronchoconstriction, hypotension, pallor, clammy skin, loss of consciousness, rapid pulse and death if adequate treatment is not administered.

2.44 BCD

Hodgkin's disease is a type of lymphoma in which lymphatic tissue is affected, often initially in the neck. Acute leukaemias account for about half of all childhood malignant diseases. Patients with leukaemias often have bleeding tendencies and increased susceptibility to infections; hence they often have bleeding gingivae. Multiple myeloma is a disseminated disease and neoplastic cells are deposited in bone marrow, accounting for the bone pain. Oral squamous cell carcinomas are usually treated with surgery and radiotherapy either independently or in combination. They are usually not treated with chemotherapy alone.

2.45 All statements are false

Antibiotic prophylaxis is no longer required for dental procedures. For more information please see www.nice.org.uk

3

Oral
Medicine

3.1 **Which of the following statements about infections are correct?**

A   Mumps is a common bacterial infection that causes bilateral enlargement of the parotid glands

B   Foot and mouth disease is caused by Coxsackie A virus and is characterised by a viral rash and oral ulceration

C   The Ebstein–Barr virus causes infectious mononucleosis, in which petechiae of the palate and ulceration of the fauces are seen

D   Primary herpetic stomatitis is caused by the herpes zoster virus, usually type 1 and is a condition in which intra-oral vesicles occur, which rapidly break down to form ulcerated areas

E   A patient with a facial palsy and vesicles of herpes zoster in the external auditory meatus is likely to have Ramsay–Hunt syndrome

3.2 **Which of the following statements are correct with respect to the salivary glands and calculi?**

A   Meal time syndrome only occurs if a patient has a blockage in salivary flow due to a salivary calculus

B   Salivary calculi form more commonly in the parotid gland than the submandibular gland

C   Encouraging salivary flow by chewing may help small salivary calculi to pass out through the salivary duct

D   Salivary calculi are more common in males than in females

E   Salivary calculi are always radiopaque due to calcium deposits, and hence are visible on radiographs

3.3 **Which of the following are well-known effects of chewing betel nut/ paan?**

A   Oral submucous fibrosis

B   Oral dysplasia

C   Oral candidiasis

D   Cervical caries

E   Fissured depapillated tongue

3.1   CE

Mumps is caused by paramyxovirus and hence is a viral infection. It does cause painful enlargement of the parotid glands but it may affect other glands as well. Hand, foot and mouth disease is caused by Coxsackie A virus and is characterised by a viral rash and oral ulceration, whereas foot and mouth disease is a disease of cattle caused by a rhinovirus. Other signs and symptoms of infectious mononucleosis are cervical lymphadenopathy, sore throat, tonsillar exudates and pyrexia.

Primary herpetic stomatitis is usually caused by the type 1 herpes simplex virus. It does cause a vesicular stomatitis, which may be accompanied by malaise, tiredness and a sore throat. Ramsay–Hunt syndrome involves herpes zoster infection affecting the geniculate ganglion, which results in facial weakness, and vesicles of zoster are seen in the ear and pharynx.

3.2   CD

Meal time syndrome occurs if a patient has any type of blockage in salivary flow (eg calculus, stricture, mucus plug, etc.) from a major gland. Eighty per cent of salivary calculi form in the submandibular gland, and it could be due to the composition of the saliva and the position and length of the duct. Salivary calculi occur most commonly in adult males. Not all salivary calculi are radiopaque, and sometimes are only visualised on further imaging, eg a sialogram.

3.3   AB

Chewing betel nut/paan is known to be a risk factor for oral submucous fibrosis, oral dysplasia and squamous cell carcinoma. Oral candidiasis, cervical caries and a fissured depapillated tongue are often caused by a dry mouth.

3.4 **Which of the following factors predispose a patient to oral and oropharyngeal squamous cell carcinoma?**

A   Smokeless tobacco use

B   Sunlight

C   Viral infection

D   Vitamin C deficiency

E   Vitamin K deficiency

3.5 **Which of the following statements are correct regarding medications used to treat various types of pain in the orofacial region?**

A   Idiopathic facial pain or atypical facial pain may be treated effectively with tricyclic antidepressants

B   Temporal arteritis may be treated effectively with clonazepam

C   Trigeminal neuralgia may be treated effectively with carbamazepine

D   Trigeminal neuralgia may be treated effectively with gabapentin

E   Post-herpetic neuralgia may be treated effectively with aciclovir

3.6 **Which of the following descriptions of the types of facial pain are correct?**

A   Myofascial pain is often poorly localised

B   Pain from internal derangement of the temporomandibular joint is usually poorly localised

C   Periodic migrainous neuralgia (cluster headache) is often associated with facial flushing on the affected side of the face

D   If a young patient is diagnosed with migrainous neuralgia (cluster headache), it may well be due to multiple sclerosis

E   Atypical facial pain (idiopathic facial pain) is often poorly localised and may occur in the absence of organic signs

3.4 ABC

The aetiology of oral squamous cell carcinoma is multifactorial and it is generally thought that the numerous risk factors include all kinds of tobacco usage, excessive alcohol usage, betel nut/paan chewing, immunodeficiency, vitamin A deficiency, chronic infections such as candidal and syphilitic infections, and oral mucosal diseases including submucous fibrosis and lichen planus. Infection with the human papilloma virus (especially HPV-16) increases the risk of oropharyngeal cancer. Sunlight is also thought to play a role in lip cancer. For further information, see the Cancer Research UK website (http://info.cancerresearchuk.org).

3.5 ACD

Temporal arteritis may be treated effectively with steroids. Post-herpetic neuralgia may be treated effectively with gabapentin or antidepressants. The initial viral infection may be effectively treated with aciclovir, but not the resultant neuralgic pain.

3.6 ACE

Pain due to internal derangement of the temporomandibular joint is usually well localised as opposed to myofascial pain, which is often poorly localised. Periodic migrainous neuralgia (cluster headache) is often associated with facial flushing, as well as a watery eye and a runny nose on the affected side. Young patients with symptoms of trigeminal neuralgia may have multiple sclerosis.

3.7 **Which of the following conditions are associated with a known increased risk of malignant change?**

A   Geographic tongue

B   Hairy leukoplakia

C   Sublingual keratosis

D   Denture stomatitis

E   Erosive lichen planus

3.8 **A patient presents with a sore mouth. Which haematological tests would you request?**

A   Full blood count (FBC)

B   Serum ferritin

C   Alkaline phosphatase levels

D   Urea and electrolytes (U&Es)

E   Mean corpuscular volume (MCV)

3.9 **Which of the following are signs of primary herpetic gingivostomatitis?**

A   Dry mouth

B   Intra-oral vesicles

C   Labial vesicles

D   Intra-oral ulcers

E   Low haemoglobin

3.7   CE

Sublingual keratosis has a higher rate of malignant transformation than normal mucosa, as does erosive lichen planus. All the other conditions do not have a higher rate of malignant change.

3.8   ABE

A sore mouth may be due to haematological deficiency and hence blood tests are indicated when a patient complains of a sore mouth. FBC is indicated to determine if the patient is anaemic. The anaemic may be secondary to iron, folate or vitamin B_{12} deficiency. MCV is indicated to determine if the anaemia is microcytic (eg iron deficiency) or macrocytic (B_{12} or folate deficiency).

3.9   BD

Primary herpetic gingivostomatitis is a viral infection caused by the herpes simplex virus. It is usually a subclinical infection. Patients have vesicles that may occur on any part of the oral mucosa, which burst leaving ulcers. Dry mouth and low haemoglobin are not usually seen in this condition. Labial vesicles are seen in recurrent herpes simplex infections.

3.10 **Which of the following are used to treat patients with primary herpetic gingivostomatitis?**

A   A broad-spectrum antibiotic

B   Analgesics

C   An anti-fungal medication

D   Fluids

E   Aciclovir

3.11 **Which of the following are features of secondary Sjögren's syndrome?**

A   Dry mouth (xerostomia)

B   Anosmia (loss of smell)

C   Connective tissue disease

D   Dry eyes (xerophthalmia)

E   Increased incidence of oral squamous cell carcinoma (SCC)

3.12 **Which of the following describes the pain of trigeminal neuralgia?**

A   Dull ache

B   Electric shock-like

C   Activated by touching a trigger zone

D   Usually prevents patients' sleeping

E   Lasts for hours

3.10 BDE

Primary herpetic gingivostomatitis is a viral infection. Therefore it is not treated with antibiotics or anti-fungals. Aciclovir can be used in severe cases and when there is widespread infection, but it needs to be given early. In milder cases bed rest, analgesics and fluids are usually sufficient

3.11 ACD

In secondary Sjögren's syndrome, either xerostomia (dry mouth) or xerophthalmia (dry eyes) occurs in association with an autoimmune connective tissue disorder. Patients do not lose their sense of smell (anosmia) or have a higher incidence of oral SCC.

3.12 BC

Trigeminal neuralgia is an intense, excruciating, paroxysmal pain, often described as a shooting or electric shock-like pain. It lasts seconds and usually occurs when a trigger zone is touched. It does not usually keep patients awake at night.

3.13 Which of the following can be used to treat trigeminal neuralgia?

A   Jaw exercises in retruded position

B   Carbamazepine

C   Baclofen

D   Phenytoin

E   Flumazenil

3.14 Which of the following drugs has gingival hyperplasia as a side effect?

A   Phenytoin

B   Carbamazepine

C   Nifedipine

D   Cisplatin

E   Ciclosporin

3.15 Which of the following conditions are strongly associated with human immunodeficiency virus (HIV) infection?

A   Kaposi's carcinoma

B   Hairy leukoplakia

C   Candidiasis

D   Lichen planus

E   Necrotising ulcerative gingivitis

3.13   BCD

Retruded jaw exercises are helpful in the management of temporomandibular joint dysfunction. Flumazenil is a benzodiazepine antagonist used for the reversal of the central sedative effects of benzodiazepines. Carbamazepine, baclofen and phenytoin may all be used for the treatment of trigeminal neuralgia.

3.14   ACE

Gingival hyperplasia is a common side effect of calcium-channel blockers such as nifedipine and diltiazem. It also occurs with phenytoin and ciclosporin.

3.15   BCE

Kaposi's sarcoma is commonly associated with HIV infection. Hairy leukoplakia is strongly associated with HIV; non-HIV cases do occur but usually in immunocompromised patients. Candidal infections are extremely common in HIV-infected patients as is periodontal disease including acute necrotising ulcerative gingivitis.

3.16 Which of the following drugs commonly cause lichenoid reactions?

    A   Gold

    B   Non-steroidal anti-inflammatory drugs (NSAIDs)

    C   β-Blockers

    D   Carbamazepine

    E   Oral hypoglycaemics

3.17 Which of the following are types of lichen planus?

    A   Reticular

    B   Erosive

    C   Pseudomembranous

    D   Bullous

    E   Hyperplastic

3.18 Which of the following are treatments options for lichen planus?

    A   No treatment

    B   Fluconazole

    C   Triamcinolone acetonide

    D   Azathioprine

    E   Pilocarpine

3.16   ABCE

Many drugs have been found to cause lichenoid reactions including anti-malarials, NSAIDs, gold, some tricyclic antidepressants, oral hypoglycaemics, methyldopa, penicillamine and β-blockers.

3.17   ABD

Six types of lichen planus have been described: reticular, papular, plaque-like, atrophic (desquamative gingivitis), erosive/ulcerative and bullous. Pseudomembranous and hyperplastic are types of candidiasis.

3.18   ACD

Treatment is not always required for lichen planus, and depends on the severity. Active treatment ranges from topical to systemic corticosteroids. In severe cases immunosuppressants, eg azathioprine and ciclosporin, may be necessary. Fluconazole is an anti-fungal used for the treatment of candidiasis. Pilocarpine is a parasympathomimetic used in the treatment of dry mouth.

3.19 **Which of the following conditions are associated with bullous lesions?**

    A   Epidermolysis bullosa

    B   Linear Ig A disease

    C   Erythema multiforme

    D   Pemphigus

    E   Bulimia

3.20 **Which of the following statements are true?**

    A   Lichen planus is characterised by mononuclear inflammatory infiltrate in the lamina propria

    B   The rate of malignant transformation with lichen planus is in the order of 10%

    C   Patients with systemic lupus erythematosus (SLE) may present with a malar rash

    D   Pemphigus is more common in children

    E   Behçet's syndrome may present with conjunctivitis and uveitis

3.21 **Which of the following are true regarding Sjögren's syndrome?**

    A   It is more common in females

    B   Primary Sjögren's may be associated with rheumatoid arthritis

    C   Autoantibodies against ribonucleotide are found: SS-A or Ro and SS-B or La

    D   May lead to B-cell lymphoma (MALTOMA)

    E   Tricyclic antidepressants may be helpful

3.19 ABD

Epidermolysis bullosa and pemphigus may present with bullous lesions, as may linear IgA disease. Bulimia presents with tooth erosion, and erythema multiforme presents with ulcers and blood-stained, crusted lips.

3.20 ACE

The rate of malignant transformation with lichen planus is in the order of 1%. Pemphigus is found mainly in middle-aged and older patients. SLE patients present with the classic malar 'butterfly' rash.

3.21 ACD

Secondary Sjögren's syndrome comprises dry eyes or dry mouth together with a connective tissue or autoimmune disease – not primary Sjögren's syndrome. Dry mouth is a side effect of tricyclic antidepressants.

3.22 Regarding aphthous ulcers:

A   They are more common in males

B   The herpetiform-type are more common in males

C   Haematinic deficiencies are detected in approximately 50% of cases

D   They can be associated with cessation of smoking

E   They are often helped by the used of antidepressants

3.23 Which of the following lesions/conditions are caused by viruses?

A   Koplik's spots

B   Herpetiform ulcers

C   Herpes labialis

D   Ramsay–Hunt syndrome

E   Lyme disease

3.24 Patients with which of the following conditions are more likely to get oral candidal infections than those without?

A   Patients undergoing chemotherapy

B   Sjögren's syndrome

C   Diabetes mellitus

D   Anaemia

E   Malnourishment

3.22   D

Aphthous ulcers are slightly commoner in females than males. Haematinic deficiencies are detected in up to 20% of patients, and the ulcers can sometimes be associated with smoking cessation. The main treatment after correction of haematinic deficiencies is topical corticosteroids.

3.23   ACD

Koplik's spots are seen in the buccal mucosa in patients with measles, which is an infection caused by paramyxovirus. Herpes labialis is caused by the herpes simplex virus and Ramsay–Hunt syndrome is due to herpes zoster of the geniculate ganglion. Herpetiform ulcers are a type of aphthous ulcer and are not caused by a virus. Lyme disease is caused by *Borrelia burgdorferi*, a spirochaetal bacterium, and is spread via ticks.

3.24   ABCDE

Candidal infections are commoner in patients with other underlying disease processes. Hence patients with anaemia, diabetes mellitus and those who are malnourished or undergoing chemotherapy are more at risk of candidal infections. Patients with Sjögren's syndrome suffer from dry mouth, which puts them at greater risk of candidal infections.

3.25 **Which of the following conditions can be associated with oral mucosal disease?**

A Crohn's disease

B Irritable bowel syndrome (IBS)

C Ulcerative colitis

D Peutz–Jeghers syndrome

E Bowen's disease

3.26 **Which of the following are treatments for dry mouth?**

A Pilocarpine

B Salivary substitutes based on carboxymethylcellulose

C Mucin-based salivary substitutes

D Atropine

E Hyoscine

3.27 **Angular cheilitis can be:**

A Caused by candidal infection of the commissures

B Caused by *Staphylococcus aureus* infection of the commissures

C Caused by an increase in occlusal vertical dimension in patients wearing dentures

D Treated with aciclovir cream

E Treated with miconazole cream

3.25 ACD

Bowen's disease is carcinoma-in-situ of the skin. Crohn's disease may affect any part of the gastrointestinal tract and hence the oral cavity may be involved. Lesions seen are cobblestoning of the buccal mucosa, glossitis, mucosal tags and swelling of the lips. In Peutz–Jeghers syndrome pigmented macules are seen around the perioral region. In ulcerative colitis, aphthous ulcers may be seen possibly due to the malabsorption which accompanies the condition. IBS is not usually associated with oral lesions.

3.26 ABC

Pilocarpine stimulates muscarinic receptors in the salivary glands and hence increases the production of saliva. It is used for patients who have some residual salivary gland function following radiotherapy. Artificial saliva may be used for symptomatic relief of dry mouth and can be based on carboxymethylcellulose or mucin. Atropine and hyoscine are anti-muscarinic drugs that dry up secretions.

3.27 ABE

Angular cheilitis is a combined staphylococcal and fungal infection that occurs at the angles of the mouth. It has been previously attributed to a decreased occlusal vertical dimension in denture wearers, but increasing the vertical dimension alone will not treat the infection. Treatment can involve fusidic acid cream and an antifungal, eg miconazole. Aciclovir is an anti-viral medication and hence not indicated for angular cheilitis.

3.28 Although the aetiology of recurrent aphthous ulceration is unknown, which of the following are thought to be associated with aphthous ulceration?

A   Smoking

B   Haematinic deficiencies

C   Stress

D   Family history

E   HIV

3.29 Which of the following oral lesions are known to be related to candidal infections?

A   Antibiotic sore mouth

B   Denture stomatitis

C   Median rhomboid glossitis

D   Geographical tongue (erythema migrans)

E   Hairy leukoplakia

3.30 Dry mouth may be caused by:

A   Hyperbaric oxygen treatment of osteoradionecrosis

B   Sjögren's syndrome

C   Sarcoidosis

D   Bell's palsy

E   Parkinson's disease

3.28 BCDE

The cause of recurrent aphthous ulceration is unknown, but several associations have been made. Stress, haematinic deficiencies and a family history all predispose a patient to getting aphthae. The ulcers also occur in HIV infections, being more severe in the more immunocompromised cases. Smoking is not associated with aphthae, in fact patients who do not smoke or who have recently stopped smoking are more likely to suffer from aphthae.

3.29 ABC

Antibiotic sore mouth and denture stomatitis are caused by candidal infection. Previously median rhomboid glossitis was thought to be a developmental condition, but it is now thought to be due to chronic atrophic candidal infection on the tongue. The cause of geographic tongue is unknown. Hairy leukoplakia occurs in HIV-infected patients and immunocompromised individuals. The lesion may be secondarily infected with *Candida*, but it is not the cause of the lesion.

3.30 BC

Bell's palsy and Parkinson's disease are commonly associated with hypersalivation (ptyalism). Hyperbaric oxygen treatment does not cause a dry mouth although the patients may have a dry mouth following the radiotherapy. Both Sjögren's syndrome and sarcoidosis may cause a dry mouth.

3.31 Regarding oral cancer:

A   It accounts for approximately 10% of cancers in the UK

B   It is commoner in men

C   Smoking and heavy alcohol intake are synergistic risk factors

D   Chewed tobacco (betel nut) is safer than smoked tobacco

E   It may arise in white patches

3.32 Which of the following are potentially malignant oral lesions?

A   Oral submucosal fibrosis

B   Speckled leukoplakia

C   Actinic cheilitis

D   Erythema migrans

E   Erythema multiforme

3.33 Regarding mucous membrane pemphigoid:

A   It is commoner in men

B   The onset is in the third to fourth decade

C   It is characterised by deposits of immunoglobulins and complement components in the basement membrane

D   It is characterised by loss of intercellular adherence of supra-basal spinous cells

E   Ocular involvement may lead to blindness

3.31 BCE

Oral cancer accounts for approximately 2% of cancers in the UK, and traditionally it was a disease of older men. However, the incidence is increasing in younger patients and women. Smoking and alcohol consumption are risk factors and are thought to act synergistically. Chewing betel nut is also a risk factor and important in the Indian subcontinent where it is commonly practised. White patches in the mouth have a potential for malignant change.

3.32 ABC

Various potentially malignant conditions occur in the oral cavity. The lesion with the highest rate of malignant transformation is erythroplasia. Speckled leukoplakia and leukoplakia also have the potential to turn malignant. Oral submucous fibrosis, lichen planus, actinic cheilitis, chronic hyperplastic candidosis and lupus erythematosus are all potentially malignant lesions.

3.33 CE

Loss of intercellular adherence of supra-basal spinous cells is characteristic of pemphigus vulgaris; in pemphigoid the split occurs at the level of the basement membrane. Mucous membrane pemphigoid is twice as common in women and usually affects people in their fifth to sixth decades. One complication of the disease is ocular involvement, which may lead to scarring and blindness.

3.34   Desquamative gingivitis is seen in which of the following conditions?

A   Lichen planus

B   Pemphigus vulgaris

C   Erythema multiforme

D   Erythema migrans

E   Mucous membrane pemphigoid

3.35   Regarding Bell's palsy:

A   It is an upper motor neurone lesion

B   It causes a unilateral paralysis of all the muscles of facial expression

C   It is thought to be due to compression of the facial nerve in the pterygomaxillary fissure

D   Loss of taste may also be associated

E   It is usually treated with low-dose steroids

3.36   Regarding herpes infections of the trigeminal area:

A   Reactivation of the herpes simplex virus usually causes cold sores on the lips

B   Herpetic whitlows can be caught only from patients with primary herpes infections

C   Post-herpetic neuralgia follows a herpes simplex infection

D   Post-herpetic neuralgia usually responds well to treatment with carbamazepine

E   Post-herpetic neuralgia usually occurs in young patients

3.34 ABE

In desquamative gingivitis, the gingivae are red, inflamed and atrophic. It occurs in lichen planus, pemphigus vulgaris and mucous membrane pemphigoid.

3.35 BD

Bell's palsy is a lower motor neurone lesion of the facial nerve, and as such it causes unilateral paralysis of all the muscles of facial expression. Upper motor neurone lesions affecting the facial nerve do not cause paralysis of the forehead as there is some cross-over in innervation. The palsy is thought to be due to compression of the facial nerve in the stylomastoid canal. Loss of taste occurs due to the chorda tympani being affected. Treatment is usually with high-dose steroids initially, which are then tailed off.

3.36 A

Reactivation of the herpes simplex virus does cause herpes labialis, which takes the form of cold sores on the lips. Herpetic whitlows can be caught from patients with primary or secondary herpetic infections. Post-herpetic neuralgia follows herpes zoster infection, and usually occurs in older people. The response to carbamazepine is often poor.

4

Oral
Pathology

4.1 **Which of the following statements regarding salivary lumps are correct?**

A   A 1 cm lump in the upper lip is most likely to be mucocoele

B   A 1 cm lump in the lower lip is most likely to be mucocoele

C   About 75% of tumours in the submandibular gland are malignant

D   About 30% of all salivary gland tumours occur in the sublingual gland and the majority of these are malignant

E   Intraoral salivary glands account for about 10% of all salivary gland tumours with about half of these being benign

4.2 **Which of the following are types of Langerhans' cells histiocytosis?**

A   Letterer–Siwe syndrome

B   Solitary eosinophilic granuloma

C   Hand–Schuller–Christian disease

D   Melkersson–Rosenthal syndrome

E   Solitary plasmacytoma

4.3 **Which of the following statements regarding biopsies are correct?**

A   When choosing the site to biopsy in a large lesion the most important consideration is to place the biopsy in the site that is likely to heal with the least amount of discomfort to the patient

B   A suture need not be placed through the tissue to be biopsied if you are using non-toothed forceps, as these will not crush the tissue and will not leave marks on the specimen

C   Sloughing or necrotic areas of tissue should be avoided

D   A commonly used fixative is 20% formal saline

E   The specimen must not be processed until it has been in the fixative for at least 24 hours

4.1 BE

A small lump in the upper lip is most likely to be a pleomorphic adenoma whereas a lump in the lower lip is most likely to be a mucocoele. About a third of tumours in the submandibular gland are malignant. About 0.3% of all salivary gland tumours occur in the sublingual gland and the majority of these are malignant.

4.2 ABC

Langerhans' cells are antigen-presenting cells present in the epithelium. If they give rise to bone tumours, three forms are recognised: Letterer–Siwe syndrome, solitary eosinophilic granuloma and multifocal eosinophilic granuloma, including Hand–Schuller–Christian disease. Melkersson–Rosenthal syndrome is a condition in which patients have facial paralysis along with chronic granulomatous lesions similar to Crohn's disease. Plasmacytoma is a tumour of plasma cells, not Langerhans' cells.

4.3 C

When choosing the site to biopsy in a large lesion the most important consideration is to select the most suspicious looking area(s). A suture should be placed through the tissue to be biopsied for several reasons: it can be used to orientate the biopsy, it can prevent it being aspirated and it prevent crush marks that can be made with any type of instrument. A commonly used fixative is 10% formal saline, which is formaldehyde solution in normal saline. The length of time it takes a specimen to fix depends on its size. Smaller specimens will fix in less than 24 hours so could be processed sooner.

4.4 **Which of the following are features of Gorlin–Goltz syndrome (basal cell carcinoma/jaw cyst syndrome)**

A Absence of clavicles

B Calcified falx cerebellum

C Frontal and parietal bossing

D Multiple dentigerous cysts

E Multiple basal cell haemangiomas

4.5 **Which of the following are microscopic features of epithelial dysplasia?**

A Atypical mitosis

B Hyperkeratinisation

C Loss of cellular polarity

D Altered nuclear/cytoplasmic ratio

E Loss or reduction of intercellular adherence

4.6 **Which of the following microscopic features are suggestive of the white lesion of lichen planus?**

A Saw tooth rete ridges

B Hypokeratosis

C Dense band of macrophages below the basement membrane

D Basal cell liquefaction

E Acantholysis

4.7 **Carcinoma of the lip:**

A Is commoner in the upper lip

B Is often caused by chewing betel nut/paan

C Has a worse prognosis than intra-oral carcinoma

D Is principally caused by alcohol consumption

E Often occurs in patients with submucous fibrosis

4.4 C

Gorlin–Goltz (basal cell carcinoma/jaw cyst) syndrome has many features including calcified falx cerebri, multiple basal cell carcinomas, skeletal abnormalities and multiple odontogenic keratocysts (keratocystic odontogenic tumours). The clavicles are absent in cleidocranial dysostosis.

4.5 ACDE

Dysplasia is a term used to describe histological abnormalities seen in both premalignant and malignant cells. Abnormal features include: abnormal mitoses and increased number of mitoses; loss of polarity; drop-shaped rete ridges; abnormal intercellular adherence; and abnormal nuclear/cytoplasmic ratio. Abnormal keratinisation occurs in cells situated more basally than in the layers in which cells normally keratinise. Hyperkeratinisation is not a feature of dysplasia.

4.6 AD

The typical histological features of lichen planus include saw tooth rete ridges, hyperkeratosis or parakeratosis, a dense band of lymphocytes below the basement membrane and basal cell liquefaction.

4.7 All statements are false

Carcinoma of the lip is commoner on the lower lip. It is often identified early because it is visible and hence has a better prognosis than intra-oral carcinoma. The main risk factor for carcinoma of the lip is exposure to sunlight, and it is not affected by alcohol consumption or betel nut chewing in the same way as intra-oral carcinoma. Intra-oral carcinoma commonly occurs in patients with submucous fibrosis.

4.8 In anhidrotic ectodermal dysplasia:

A There are often supernumerary teeth

B Hair is usually scanty

C A sex-linked recessive trait is usually the cause

D Anhidrosis refers to the type of hair present

E Teeth are often peg shaped

4.9 Delayed eruption of teeth is a feature of which of the following conditions?

A Cleidocranial dysostosis

B Osteogenesis imperfecta

C Rickets

D Cherubism

E Scurvy

4.10 Regarding dental fluorosis:

A It affects deciduous teeth and permanent teeth equally

B It causes white or brownish mottling of teeth

C Mottled teeth are less susceptible to caries than teeth not exposed to fluoride

D It occurs in areas when fluoride in the drinking water exceeds 1 ppm

E It occurs in areas when fluoride in the drinking water exceeds 2 ppm

4.8 BCE

Anhidrotic ectodermal dysplasia is usually a sex-linked recessive trait that results in hypodontia, hypotrichosis (scanty and wispy hair) and anhidrosis (inability to sweat). Any teeth present are often peg shaped or conical.

4.9 ACD

Delayed eruption of teeth usually occurs in cleidocranial dysostosis and rickets. In cherubism eruption may be delayed due to displacement by the giant cell lesions.

4.10 BCE

Excess fluoride ingestion causes dental fluorosis. Fluoride is usually present in drinking water and effects are seen when it exceeds 2 ppm. Mottling of the teeth occurs and appears as white or brown areas on the teeth with varying degrees of pitting. Permanent teeth are usually affected – it rarely affects deciduous teeth.

4.11 Regarding dental caries:

A   Lactobacilli are the bacteria that are the main cause of dental caries

B   Cariogenic bacteria produce acid

C   Glucose is more cariogenic than sucrose

D   Fructose is less cariogenic than sucrose

E   Sugar alcohols (polyols) are cariogenic

4.12 Acute osteomyelitis:

A   Affects the maxilla more commonly than the mandible

B   Always causes paraesthesia in relation to the inferior dental nerve

C   Will not be apparent on radiographs until about 10 days

D   Usually causes sharp, shooting pain

E   May cause associated teeth to loosen

4.13 Regarding actinomycosis:

A   It is a suppurative infection caused by a coccal bacterium, usually *Actinomyces israelii*

B   It is more common in women than men

C   It usually affects middle-aged people

D   Multiple discharging sinuses are seen, and the pus contains 'sulphur granules' (bacterial colonies)

E   It is treated with metronidazole

4.11   BD

Viridans streptococci are the most cariogenic bacteria and not lactobacilli, which tend to appear in bacterial plaque after caries has developed. All cariogenic bacteria produce acid. The most cariogenic sugar is sucrose – both glucose and fructose are less cariogenic than sucrose. Sugar alcohols are non-cariogenic and so are used in 'sugar-free' foods.

4.12   CE

Acute osteomyelitis commonly affects the mandible. Osteomyelitis of the maxilla is rare although it may occur in infants. Acute osteomyelitis is associated with severe, deep-seated, throbbing pain, the associated teeth become tender and loose, and pus may exude from the socket. Alteration in sensation in relation to the inferior dental nerve may occur, but not in all cases.

Radiographic changes are not visible initially, only becoming apparent after about 10 days, when loss of trabeculae and areas of bone destruction are evident.

4.13   CD

Actinomycosis is a suppurative infection that is usually caused by *Actinomyces israelii*, a filamentous bacterium. It most commonly tends to affect men aged about 30–60 years. Multiple discharging sinuses are seen, and the pus contains granules known as 'sulphur granules', which are colonies of *Actinomyces* species. Treatment involves drainage of the pus along with penicillin or tetracycline.

4.14   Regarding radicular cysts:

A   The cyst capsule often contains cholesterol crystals

B   The cyst fluid often shimmers due to the keratin contained within

C   The cyst lining is formed of stratified squamous epithelium

D   Rushton's bodies in the cyst wall indicate that the cyst is actively growing

E   Radicular cysts are always associated with a non-vital pulp

4.15   Keratocysts (keratocystic odontogenic tumours):

A   Are always multilocular

B   Are commoner in the mandible than the maxilla

C   Grow along the bone rather than expanding the jaw

D   Are always associated with a missing tooth

E   Commonly recur

4.16   Patients with Gorlin–Goltz syndrome (or basal cell carcinoma/jaw cyst syndrome) have:

A   Multiple radicular cysts

B   Frontal and parietal bossing

C   Multiple basal cell carcinomas of the skin

D   Supernumerary teeth

E   Skeletal abnormalities such as bifid ribs and vertebral abnormalities

4.14   ACE

Radicular cysts are formed following infection or inflammation of the pulp and are associated with non-vital roots. The cyst lining is formed of stratified squamous epithelium, which contains hyaline or Rushton's bodies, which indicate the odontogenic origin of the cyst. The cyst capsule contains cholesterol crystals and the cholesterol in the cyst fluid gives it a shimmering appearance.

4.15   BCE

Keratocysts (keratocystic odontogenic tumours) are often unilocular when small and become multilocular as they enlarge. They are thought to be formed from the remnants of the dental lamina and so are not always associated with a missing tooth. They are commoner in the mandible than the maxilla. They commonly recur due to the difficulty of removing all of the friable lining.

4.16   BCE

The features of Gorlin–Goltz syndrome are multiple keratocysts (keratocystic odontogenic tumours), multiple basal cell carcinomas, intra-cranial abnormalities such as calcification of the falx cerebri, and frontal bossing and other skeletal abnormalities including bifid ribs.

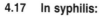

4.17 **In syphilis:**

    A A primary chancre in the oral cavity may appear about 3–4 weeks after infection

    B The primary chancre is also known as a snail track ulcer

    C The primary chancre often heals after 2 months with severe scarring

    D The secondary stage usually occurs 1–4 months after the primary infection

    E The tertiary stage involves the appearance of well-defined, rounded areas known as mucous patches

4.18 **Hairy leukoplakia:**

    A Only ever occurs in human immunodeficiency virus (HIV)-positive patients

    B Is caused by candidal infection of the oral mucosa

    C Commonly affects the dorsum of the tongue

    D Is a premalignant condition

    E Has koilocyte-like cells in the prickle cell layer

4.19 **Regarding an oral dysplastic lesion:**

    A It should be managed with 6-monthly check-up at the dentist

    B Stop any habits that may be contributory, eg smoking, alcohol consumption

    C Surgical removal of the whole dysplastic area

    D Leukoplakias have a higher risk of malignant transformation than erythroplasia

    E High-risk sites include the hard palate

4.17   AD

An oral chancre appears in primary syphilis about 3–4 weeks after infection. It often heals without scarring after a couple of months. In secondary syphilis the oral lesions consist of ulcers that are covered with a greyish slough known as snail track ulcers. When ulcers join together, larger areas are involved and these are known as mucous patches. The lesion in tertiary syphilis is the gumma.

4.18   E

Hairy leukoplakia occurs most commonly in homosexual men infected with HIV. It also occurs in immunodeficient patients although it is not as common. It is often secondarily infected with *Candida*, and occurs most commonly on the lateral borders of the tongue. It is not a premalignant condition. Histologically there is hyperkeratosis or parakeratosis. In the prickle cell layer are vacuolated and ballooned cells with dark nuclei surrounded by a clear halo – koilocyte-like cells.

4.19   B

Dysplastic lesions should be reviewed 3 months after elimination of risk factors and regularly thereafter. Surgical excision of the lesion may be indicated if the lesion persists, depending on the degree of dysplasia, and site and extent of the lesion. Erythroplasia (erythroplakia) and non-homogeneous leukoplakias have a much higher risk of malignant transformation than homogeneous leukoplakias. The high-risk sites include the ventrolateral surfaces of the tongue, floor of the mouth and soft palate/fauces.

4.20 Salivary calculi:

A Commonly cause dry mouth

B Occur most commonly in the sublingual gland

C Occur most commonly in the parotid gland

D Are always visible on radiographs

E May be asymptomatic

4.21 With respect to salivary gland tumours:

A About 75% of all salivary gland tumours occur in the parotid gland

B About 10% of all salivary gland tumours occur in the minor salivary glands

C A tumour in the parotid gland is more likely to be malignant than a tumour in the minor salivary glands

D Most tumours in the sublingual salivary gland are benign

E The commonest salivary gland tumour is a adenoid cystic carcinoma

4.22 With respect to salivary gland tumours:

A Pleomorphic adenomas usually undergo malignant change

B Pleomorphic adenomas may contain fibrous, myxoid and elastic tissue

C Mucoepidermoid carcinomas have a characteristic 'Swiss cheese' pattern

D Acinic cell carcinomas commonly spread along nerve sheaths

E Adenoid cystic carcinomas have a poor prognosis

4.20   E

Salivary calculi occur most commonly in the submandibular gland and may be asymptomatic. They are not always visible on radiographs and do not cause a dry mouth.

4.21   AB

About three-quarters of all salivary gland tumours occur in the parotid gland, and about a tenth occur in the minor salivary glands. A tumour in a minor gland is more likely to be malignant as about a third are malignant, whereas in the parotid gland only about 15% are malignant. However, a tumour in the sublingual gland is most likely to be malignant as over 80% of tumours in this site are malignant. The commonest salivary gland tumour is the pleomorphic adenoma.

4.22   BE

Only about 2–4% of pleomorphic adenomas undergo malignant change. They may contain a wide variety of tissue types including fibrous, myxoid and elastic. The characteristic 'Swiss cheese' appearance and spread along nerve sheaths is seen in adenoid cystic carcinomas. Adenoid cystic carcinomas grow slowly, metastasise late, and have a poor prognosis.

4.23 **Which of the following investigations are appropriate for the lesions?**

  A   Incisional biopsy for a suspected squamous cell carcinoma

  B   Incisional biopsy for a suspected haemangioma

  C   Excisional biopsy for a suspected fibroepithelial polyp

  D   Excisional biopsy for a white patch of unknown origin

  E   Incisional biopsy for a mucous extravasation cyst

4.24 **Regarding ameloblastoma:**

  A   It usually presents between the ages of 15 and 20 years

  B   It is the commonest odontogenic neoplasm

  C   It presents as a monolocular cyst on radiographs

  D   It is common in the posterior mandible

  E   Follicular ameloblastoma is the commonest type

4.25 **With respect to fibrous dysplasia:**

  A   It is commoner in females

  B   It typically affects the maxilla

  C   It is painful

  D   Histologically there is irregular resorption and deposition of bone

  E   Commonly occurs in the fourth decade

4.23   AC

Incisional biopsies should be done on squamous cell carcinomas and white patches of unknown origin. An excisional biopsy is appropriate for a fibroepithelial polyp and a mucous extravasation cyst. Biopsy should not be attempted on a suspected haemangioma.

4.24   BDE

Ameloblastoma usually presents between the ages of 30 and 50 years, and it presents as a multilocular cyst. The other types of ameloblastoma are: plexiform, acanthomatous, basal cell and granular cell. Unicystic ameloblastomas are considered as a distinct entity to the solid variants of ameloblastoma.

4.25   AB

In fibrous dysplasia normal bone is replaced by fibrous tissue. It usually affects the maxilla and people below the age of 20. It is not often painful. Irregular resorption and deposition of bone is seen in Paget's disease.

4.26 With respect to osteosarcoma:

    A   It is a complication of Paget's disease

    B   It is commoner in the maxilla

    C   Paraesthesia may be the presenting feature

    D   It is commoner in males

    E   It is most commonly seen in children

4.27 Regarding hyperparathyroidism:

    A   It is characterised by raised plasma calcium levels

    B   It presents with giant cell lesions

    C   Jaw lesions are commonly present

    D   Patients may present with enlargement of the skull

    E   It is most commonly secondary to chronic renal failure (CRF)

4.28 Which of the following are true of cherubism?

    A   It is a rare genetic defect of osteoclastic activity

    B   It is commoner in males

    C   The middle third of the face is usually hypoplastic

    D   Presents with lesions also known as Brown's tumours

    E   Regression of the disease occurs

4.26   ACD

Osteosarcoma is rare and more common in the mandible. It is most commonly seen between the ages of 30 and 40 years and in males. It occurs as a complication of Paget's disease, although it is not common.

4.27   ABE

Skull enlargement occurs with Paget's disease. Osteolytic lesions in bone are more commonly the result of secondary hyperparathyroidism (eg CRF) than primary (hyperplasia or adenoma of parathyroids).

4.28   ABE

Cherubism is inherited as an autosomal dominant trait. It presents with expansion of the maxilla. Brown tumours are seen secondary to hyperparathyroidism.

4.29 **Which of the following are potentially malignant oral lesions/ conditions?**

A Speckled leukoplakia

B Tertiary syphilis

C Paterson–Kelly syndrome

D Chronic candidiasis

E Medium rhomboid glossitis

4.30 **Regarding Warthin's tumour (adenolymphoma):**

A It is commoner in males

B Tall columnar eosinophilic cells covering lymphoid tissue is the characteristic histological appearance

C It is the commonest type of salivary tumour

D Average age of presentation is 40 years

E 10% are bilateral

4.31 **Which of the following features would raise suspicion of a malignant salivary tumour?**

A Facial nerve palsy

B Soft rubbery consistency

C Sudden increase in size

D Lesion is in a minor salivary gland rather than in the parotid

E Skin ulceration

4.29   ABCD

Various potentially malignant conditions occur in the oral cavity including erythroplasia, dysplastic and speckled leuokplakia, oral submucous fibrosis, tertiary syphilis, chronic candidiasis and lichen planus. There is also high incidence of oral and oesophageal cancer in Paterson–Kelly syndrome. Median rhomboid glossitis is not a potentially malignant lesion.

4.30   ABE

The male to female ratio of occurrence of Warthin's tumour is 7:1. It is a benign tumour, making up 7–8% of salivary tumours. The average age of presentation is 70 years; 40 years is the average age for presentation of pleomorphic adenomas.

4.31   ACDE

A mass of hard consistency is more likely to be malignant. Sudden increase in size of a salivary mass, even if it has been present for many years, should alert the clinician to a risk of malignant mass. Pain, nerve involvement and nodal metastases are also signs of malignant growth.

4.32 Which of the following are true of oral submucous fibrosis:

A   It is associated with smoking

B   It is at risk of malignant transformation

C   It is managed by topical corticosteroids

D   It characteristically affects the buccal mucosa

E   It may present with trismus

4.33 Regarding odontomes:

A   They are hamartomas

B   They usually present around the age of 30 years

C   They can undergo malignant transformation

D   They most commonly present in the anterior maxilla

E   The lesion is composed of cementum embedded in fibrous tissue and a surrounding capsule

4.34 Which of the following statements are true?

A   Ameloblastic fibromas usually present around the age of 50 years

B   Ghost and ameloblastic cells are characteristically seen in ameloblastic fibromas

C   Calcifying epithelial odontogenic tumour is also known as Pindborg's tumour

D   Calcifying epithelial odontogenic tumours are locally invasive

E   Adenomatoid odontogenic tumours most commonly present in the anterior maxilla

4.32 BDE

Oral submucous fibrosis is associated with betel quid chewing (smokeless tobacco). Intra-lesional injections of steroids have been tried, but the benefit is limited. The risk of malignant transformation is reported to be around 5–8%.

4.33 AD

Odontomes usually present between the ages of 10 and 20 years, and are benign lesions. They most commonly present in the anterior maxilla and posterior mandible. The lesion is composed of pulp, dentine, enamel and cementum.

4.34 CDE

Ameloblastic fibromas usually present in children or young adults. Ghost and ameloblastic cells are seen in calcifying odontogenic cysts.

5

Oral
Surgery

5.1 Which of the following drugs would put a patient at risk of developing osteonecrosis of the jaws following a tooth extraction?

A Alendronic acid

B Alfentanil

C Aldactone

D Almotriptan

E Alverine

5.2 Which of the following parameters should be routinely monitored when a patient is undergoing conscious sedation with an intravenous benzodiazepine?

A Level of consciousness

B O_2 saturation

C Pain level

D Pupillary reaction

E Verbal response

5.3 Which of the following statements are correct?

A A ranula is a mucous extravasation cyst of the sublingual gland

B A ranula often occurs after removal of a blockage in the duct of a gland

C A ranula that spreads into the submasseteric space is called a plunging ranula

D Surgical removal of a ranula may damage the lingual nerve

E Surgical removal of the ranula alone often results in recurrence so removal of the gland is often indicated

5.1   A

Alendronic acid is an oral bisphosphonate. Bisphosphonates affect bone metabolism by inhibiting osteoclast activity. Patients taking bisphosphonates are more at risk of osteonecrosis of the jaws following dental extractions as normal bony remodelling does not take place. The risk is greater with more potent bisphosphonates and those administered via an intra-venous route.

Alfentanil is a potent opioid analgesic often used for short operative procedures and day case operating due to its rapid onset of action and short duration of action. Aldactone is an aldosterone antagonist used to treat oedema and ascites in cirrhosis of the liver and congestive heart failure. Almotriptan is a 5-hydroxytryptamine agonist used to treat acute migraine. Alverine is a smooth muscle relaxant that is used to treat gastro-intestinal disorders characterised by smooth muscle spasm.

5.2   ABE

It is necessary to monitor and record a patient's level of responsiveness, airway, respiration, pulse and colour at all times when carrying out intravenous sedation. All members of the dental team must be capable of monitoring the condition of the patient and this includes pulse oximetry and blood pressure monitoring. Normal practice is to have a pulse oximeter with an alarm on it on the patient's finger at all times, and to monitor the saturation level.

It is also normal practice to maintain some degree of conversation with patients to establish their verbal response and level of consciousness throughout the procedure. Changes in pupillary response occur late in loss of consciousness and alterations here would not alert the operator to decreasing level of consciousness.

5.3   ADE

A ranula is a mucous extravasation cyst of the sublingual gland. When it extends through the mylohyoid muscle into the submental/submandibular space(s) it may appear as a neck swelling and is known as a plunging ranula.

5.4 **A patient taking warfarin attends your dental practice for extraction of a lower first permanent molar tooth. When would be an appropriate time to check his international normalised ratio (INR)?**

A At the consultation a week before the extraction

B 70 hours prior to the extraction

C 24 hours prior to the extraction

D 12 hours prior to the extraction

E An hour before the extraction

5.5 **Which of the following statements regarding oral squamous cell carcinoma in the UK are correct?**

A The incidence of lip cancer is as about the same as the incidence of tongue cancer

B The 5-year survival rate for patients with lip cancer is the better than the 5-year survival rate for those with tongue cancer in females but not in males

C The incidence of oral cancer in females is greater than that in males

D The 2-year survival rates for patients with stage I and stage II oral cancer are the same

E Overall females have a slightly better survival rate for oral cancer than males

5.6 **A patient requires a lower first permanent molar tooth to be extracted. Their medical history reveals that they have idiopathic thrombocytopenic purpura. Which of the following should be carried out to minimise the risk of complications associated with the procedure?**

A The patient should be given desmopressin (DDAVP) prior to the extraction

B The patient should have their factor IX levels measured and be given the appropriate amount of factor IX before the extraction

C The patient should have a full blood count and be given platelets if necessary

D The patient should be given intramuscular tranexamic acid prior to the extraction

E The patient must have their international normalised ratio (INR) checked within 72 hours of the extraction and the socket should be packed with a haemostatic agent and sutured

5.4 BCDE

As warfarin has a long half life it is acceptable to check the INR up to 72 hours prior to the extraction. However, the closer to the extraction time that the INR is checked the more accurate the reading. For more information, see the National Patient Safety Agency (NPSA) website (www.npsa.nhs.uk).

5.5 E

There are over four times as many tongue squamous cell carcinomas (SCCs) as there are lip SCCs within the UK, and the 5-year survival rate for lip cancer for both sexes is over 80% and for tongue it is about 40%. At present oral cancer rates in males are still greater than females although the incidence is rising in females. The 2-year survival rate for patients with stage I cancer is around 70% and for stage II oral cancer it is around 50%. (All data taken from Cancer Research UK: http://info.cancerresearchuk.org/cancerstats/types/oral/)

5.6 C

Idiopathic thrombocytopenic purpura is a disorder in which there is increased destruction of platelets so platelet numbers are reduced. Dental extractions can cause excessive bleeding so platelet levels should be assessed by a full blood count and platelet transfusion may be necessary prior to the extraction. Packing of the socket with a haemostatic agent and suturing are often carried out as well.

Desmopressin will stimulate release of factor VIIIC (endogenous pro-coagulant) and von Willebrand factor into the blood and is used for mild haemophilia A. Factor IX levels will give not information about platelet disorders, nor will measuring a patient's INR, as this measures a patient's prothrombin time against a standard prothrombin time.

Tranexamic acid is sometimes administered prior to surgery in patients with severe bleeding disorders, however it is usually administered intravenously. It can also be used as a mouthwash post extraction to help with haemostasis.

5.7   **According to the National Institute for Health and Clinical Excellence (NICE) guidelines, which of the following are indications for the removal of a lower third molar tooth?**

A   Crowding of lower anterior teeth

B   Single episode of mild pericoronitis

C   A contralateral tooth requiring removal under general anaesthetic

D   Treatment of facial pain

E   Mesioangular impaction

5.8   **Which of the following statements regarding cranial nerves are true?**

A   The abducent nerve supplies the superior oblique muscle

B   The motor supply to the muscles of mastication comes from the facial nerve

C   Sensation and taste to the posterior third of the tongue are supplied by the hypoglossal nerve

D   The trigeminal nerve is motor to the muscles of mastication

E   The lower face has bilateral facial nerve innervation

5.9   **Temporal arteritis:**

A   May cause blindness

B   Is commoner in women

C   Is treated with non-steroidal anti-inflammatory drugs (NSAIDs)

D   Results in a lowered erythrocyte sedimentation rate (ESR)

E   Causes pain in the face

5.7   All statements are false

The NICE guidelines for the removal of wisdom teeth state that none of the above are indications for removal of lower third molars. A single episode of pericoronitis could be an indication – provided that it is a severe episode.

5.8   D

The abducent nerve supplies the lateral rectus muscle of the eye; the superior oblique muscle is supplied by the trochlear nerve. The motor supply to the muscles of mastication comes from the trigeminal nerve whereas the facial nerve is motor to the muscles of facial expression. The hypoglossal nerve is motor to all the muscles of the tongue (except palatoglossus), and the glossopharyngeal nerve supplies the sensory supply to the posterior third of the tongue. The lower face has unilateral facial nerve innervation, whereas the upper face is bilaterally innervated.

5.9   ABE

Temporal arteritis or giant cell arteritis may cause blindness. It is commoner in women and results in a raised ESR, causes facial pain and is usually treated with steroids.

5.10 Which of the following muscles open(s) the mouth?

A Masseter muscle

B Temporalis muscle

C Lateral pterygoid muscle

D Digastric muscle

E Medial pterygoid muscle

5.11 Deviation of the mandible on opening could be due to:

A A unilateral anteriorly displaced disc

B Ankylosis of one condyle

C An occlusal interference between the retruded contact position (RCP) and intercuspal position (ICP)

D Internal derangement of the temporomandibular joint (TMJ)

E A fractured condyle

5.12 Cluster headache:

A Is more common in males

B Usually affects patients > 50 years of age

C May be associated with nasal congestion, watering of the eyes and facial flushing

D Can only be treated with ergotamine

E Is usually diagnosed with a computed tomography (CT) or magnetic resonance imaging (MRI) scan

5.10 CD

The masseter and medial pterygoid muscles close the mouth, as do the anterior fibres of the temporalis muscle. The lateral pterygoid and digastric muscles both open the mouth.

5.11 ABDE

Any interference with normal condylar movement may cause the mandible to deviate on opening. If the interference is on one side then the mandible usually deviates towards that side on opening as the condyle is unable to translate forward, whilst the condyle on the normal side translates forward. Occlusal interferences do not usually interfere with mandibular opening, but with closing.

5.12 AC

Cluster headache (alarm clock headache) is an intense pain centred over the temporal and eye region. There is parasympathetic activity, as the headache is often associated with facial flushing and sweating, lacrimation and rhinorrhoea, as well as ptosis and nasal congestion. It is commoner in males, usually younger than 50 years. Diagnosis is usually made on the basis of the history, although imaging may be done to rule out pathology. Treatment is symptomatic, with 'triptans' which are 5-hydroxytryptamine (5-HT) agonists or ergot alkaloids.

5.13 Glossopharyngeal neuralgia:

   A   Is more common that trigeminal neuralgia

   B   Is usually described as a dull ache

   C   May be felt in the ear on the affected side

   D   Affects the postero-lateral side of the tongue

   E   Is easily amenable to cryotherapy of the nerve

5.14 Regarding the maxillary sinus:

   A   It is not present at birth

   B   In adults it is pyramidal in shape with the base lying medially

   C   It drains via the ostium into the inferior meatus of the nose

   D   It is lined by pseudostratified ciliated columnar epithelium

   E   It is the largest of the paranasal sinuses

5.15 Osteoradionecrosis (or irradiation osteomyelitis):

   A   Is a suppurative type of osteomyelitis

   B   Affects the maxilla more commonly than the mandible

   C   Occurs due to a reduction in vascularity secondary to endarteritis
       obliterans

   D   Can occur following hyperbaric oxygen treatment for squamous cell
       carcinoma

   E   Is the same as focal sclerosing osteomyelitis

5.13 CD

Glossopharyngeal neuralgia is rare, but has the same intensity as paroxysmal trigeminal neuralgia. It may be felt in the ear as well as on the posterior third of the tongue. As the glossopharyngeal nerve is difficult to access, the condition is not amenable to cryotherapy.

5.14 BDE

The maxillary sinus is the first of the paranasal sinuses to develop and is approximately 1 cm in diameter at birth. It is pyramidal in shape with its base lying medially, forming the lateral wall of the nose. It drains via the ostium into the middle meatus of the nose.

5.15 C

Osteoradionecrosis occurs following radiotherapy to the jaws. It occurs as the bone becomes less vascular and hypocellular after the radiation treatment. It usually affects the mandible more than the maxilla. It is not caused by treatment with hyperbaric oxygen, but hyperbaric oxygen is often used to treat it. It is not a suppurating type of osteomyelitis. Focal sclerosing osteomyelitis is a rare condition thought to be due to a reaction to a low-grade infection that usually affects children and young adults. It is a different entity from osteoradionecrosis.

5.16 **In the TMN classification system:**

A   A 1.5 cm tumour on the lateral border of the tongue with no palpable neck nodes would be classified as stage 1

B   Stages are based solely on histopathological grades

C   The N classification relates only to lymph nodes on the ipsilateral side to the tumour

D   Nx means that the patient has undergone a previous neck dissection

E   M1 means distant metastasis

5.17 **The submandibular gland:**

A   Is the largest of the salivary glands

B   Empties via Stensen's duct

C   Has a duct that is closely related to the lingual nerve

D   Is the gland most commonly affected by salivary gland calculi

E   Is a mixed salivary gland

5.16   AE

The TMN (*T*umour, *N*ode, *M*etastasis) is a clinical and pathological classification system used in cancer cases. The classification is shown below.

Primary tumour	T	
	Tx	Primary tumour cannot be assessed
	T0	No evidence of primary tumour
	Tis	Carcinoma in situ
	T1	Tumour < 2 cm
	T2	Tumour 2–4 cm
	T3	Tumour > 4 cm
	T4	Tumour invades adjacent structures
Lymph nodes	N	
	Nx	Regional nodes cannot be assessed
	N0	No regional node metastasis
	N1	Metastasis in a single ipsilateral lymph node < 3 cm
	N2	Metastasis in: a single ipsilateral lymph node 3–6 cm
		in multiple ipsilateral nodes < 6 cm
		bilateral or contralateral nodes < 6 cm
	N3	Metastasis in node > 6 cm
Distant metastasis	M	
	Mx	Metastasis cannot be assessed
	M0	No distant metastasis
	M1	Distant metastasis

The stage of disease can be determined from the TNM classification as shown in the following table.

Stage	T level	N level	M level
0	Tis	N0	M0
I	T1	N0	M0
II	T2	N0	M0
III	T3	N0	M0
	T1/2	N1	M0
IV	T4	N0/1	M0
	Any T	N2/3	M0
	Any T	Any N	M1

5.17   CDE

The parotid is the largest salivary gland and it empties via Stensen's duct. The submandibular duct empties via Wharton's duct. The lingual nerve loops underneath Wharton's duct at the posterior aspect of the floor of the mouth. In this position it can easily be damaged during surgery for removing stones. The submandibular salivary gland is a mixed salivary gland and is the gland most commonly affected by salivary calculi.

5.18   Dry mouth:

   A   Can be caused by radiation therapy

   B   Can occur in diabetes mellitus

   C   Can occur with anxiety

   D   Occurs when the salivary flow rate falls below the normal of 1 ml/min

   E   Can result in an increase in root caries

5.19   Burning mouth syndrome (oral dysaesthesia, glossodynia):

   A   Is more common in females than males

   B   Usually affects patients over 50 years of age

   C   May occur in patients who are stressed or depressed

   D   Is always associated with vitamin B_1 deficiency

   E   May respond to treatment with antidepressant drugs

5.20   The lesion in the figure below is likely to be:

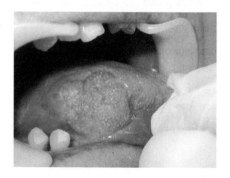

   A   Erythema migrans

   B   Median rhomboid glossitis

   C   Basal cell carcinoma

   D   Squamous cell carcinoma

   E   Traumatic ulcer

5.18   ABCE

Diabetes mellitus, irradiation therapy and anxiety can all lead to a dry mouth. It occurs when the salivary flow rate falls below 0.1 ml/min. Dry mouth may result in increased incidence of root caries.

5.19   ABCE

Burning mouth syndrome usually affects middle-aged to older women. No physical abnormality is seen. It often occurs in depressed and stressed individuals and as such responds to antidepressive drugs. Haematinic deficiencies may cause burning sensations in the oral cavity, and so should always be investigated in patients complaining of a burning mouth. If found and corrected, the burning sensation should disappear, and as such this is not burning mouth syndrome.

5.20   D

This picture shows an ulcerated area on the lateral border of the tongue. The ulcer is raised with rolled margins. Squamous cell carcinomas of the tongue may present as an ulcer with raised rolled edges. The ulcers are firm to the touch and fixed to surrounding tissue. Erythema migrans (geographical tongue) is seen as smooth red areas on the dorsum of the tongue. Medial rhomboid glossitis is as the name suggests in the mid line of the dorsum of the tongue. Basal cell carcinomas are skin lesions. Traumatic ulcers do not have a raised rolled edge and are often covered in a yellowish slough.

5.21 The appropriate management of the lesion shown in Q 5.20 may involve:

  A Incisional biopsy

  B Fine needle aspirate

  C Smear for *Candida*

  D Excisional biopsy

  E Full blood count to rule out haematinic deficiencies as the cause of the oral lesion

5.22 Identify the instruments labelled i–v in the figure. Choose from the list of options below.

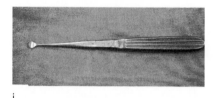

i

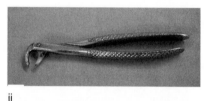

ii

iii

iv

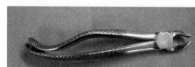

v

  A i is a Howarth's periosteal elevator

  B ii is a Kilner cheek retractor

  C iii is a pair of lower molar forceps

  D iv is a pair of bayonet forceps

  E v is a pair of upper left molar forceps

5.21 A

The appropriate management of a suspected oral squamous cell carcinoma is an incisional biopsy.

5.22 BCD

i is a Ward's periosteal elevator, iv is a pair of bayonet forceps used for extracting upper third molar teeth. v is a pair of upper molar forceps for the right not the left, (remember the beak on the forceps goes towards the cheek.)

5.23 **Identify the instruments labelled i–v in the figure. Choose from the list of options below.**

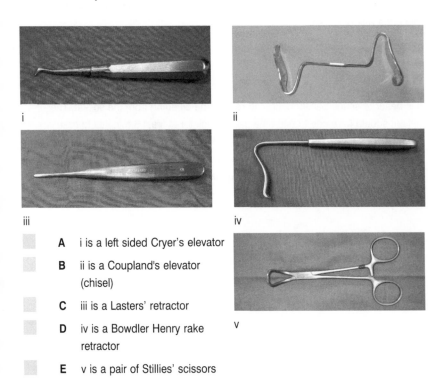

i

ii

iii

iv

v

A   i is a left sided Cryer's elevator

B   ii is a Coupland's elevator (chisel)

C   iii is a Lasters' retractor

D   iv is a Bowdler Henry rake retractor

E   v is a pair of Stillies' scissors

5.24 **You performed an extraction 3 hours earlier on a fit and healthy patient. The patient has returned to the surgery complaining of bleeding from the extraction site. The appropriate management options are:**

A   Lie the patient in the chair to calm them down

B   Get the patient to bite on a gauze pack

C   Pack the socket with Alvogyl®

D   Pack the socket with an oxidised cellulose dressing (eg Surgicel®)

E   Suture the socket using Prolene sutures

5.23 AD

ii is a straight Warwick James' elevator. iii is a Ward's buccal retractor and v is a towel clip not a pair of scissors.

5.24 BD

It is better to sit the patient upright to reduce the bleeding from the socket. The patient should be made to bite on a gauze pack for at least 5 minutes to assess the effect of continuous pressure on the socket. An appropriate dressing is oxidised cellulose (Surgicel®); Alvogyl® is used for dry sockets. The socket may need to be sutured but Prolene is not the best suture material to use in the mouth because it is a monofilament material and the cut ends are sharp. A braided alternative is better.

5.25 **You are about to extract an upper first permanent molar in a patient who has a large maxillary sinus. What should you warn the patient about prior to the extraction?**

A   Possibility of an oronasal communication

B   Possibility of an oronasal fistula

C   Possible infection following the extraction

D   Possible pain following the extraction

E   Possibility of a nose bleed following the extraction

5.26 **You are seeing a patient with an odontogenic infection. Which of the following factors would indicate that this is a severe infection which will require admission to hospital?**

A   Temperature of 38.5 °C

B   Previous episode of pain

C   Severe pain

D   Tachycardia

E   Raised floor of mouth

5.25 CD

Extraction of an upper first permanent molar in a patient with a large maxillary sinus may result in an oro-antral communication which over time may become epithelialised to form an oro-antral fistula. There is always a possibility of pain and infection after any extraction. There is no need to warn patients of nose bleeds following extractions.

5.26 ADE

Severe odontogenic infections may require hospital admission for treatment. A temperature of 38.5 °C, tachycardia and a raised floor of mouth are all indicators of a severe infection that needs in-patient treatment, so patients with these signs should all be admitted. Pain is not a good indicator of the severity of infection and hence not a good guide to whether a patient needs admission.

5.27 **To which of the following spaces can infection directly spread from a lower wisdom tooth?**

A Submasseteric space

B Pterygomaxillary space

C Submandibular space

D Cavernous sinus

E Maxillary sinus

5.28 **This radiograph shows:**

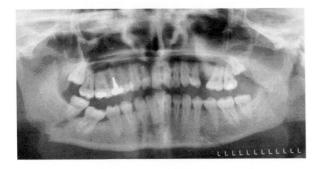

A a unilateral fractured left condyle

B a "guardsman" type fracture

C a bilateral fractured mandible

D a left mandibular body fracture

E a left mandibular angle fracture

5.29 **Which method(s) of treatment are appropriate for reduction of a fractured mandibular angle in a dentate patient:**

A Intramaxillary fixation (IMF) using eyelet wires

B IMF using arch bars

C IMF using Gunning splints

D Mini bone plates

E IMF using K-wires

5.27 ABC

Infection from a lower wisdom tooth may spread directly to the submasseteric, pterygomaxillary and submandibular spaces. Spread to the cavernous sinus is usually from infections in the middle third of the face. Infection does not spread to the maxillary sinus from lower wisdom teeth.

5.28 CD

This is a dental panoramic radiograph showing a bilateral fractured mandible. One fracture is through the right angle and the other through the left body of the mandible. The condyles appear intact with this view. A "guardsman's" fracture involves bilateral fractured condyles with a symphyseal fracture.

5.29 ABD

IMF is used for fracture reduction, so eyelet wiring and arch bars can be used for mandibular fracture reduction. Previously IMF was left on for 4–6 weeks as a means of fixation until the fracture had healed. Nowadays IMF is used during the operation to achieve the appropriate occlusion but the fracture is fixed with a mini bone plate, and the IMF is released. Gunning splints help achieve IMF in edentulous patients. K-wires are not used for IMF.

5.30 **Which of the following are well-recognised complications of removal of lower wisdom teeth?**

    A   Paraesthesia of the lingual nerve

    B   Dry socket

    C   Anaesthesia of the inferior dental nerve

    D   Paraesthesia of the inferior dental nerve

    E   Paralysis of the lingual nerve

5.31 **What are the advantages of marsupialisation of cysts compared with enucleation?**

    A   Cyst cavity open to inspection

    B   Whole cyst lining available for histological analysis

    C   Easier for the patient to look after in terms of oral hygiene

    D   May be used to prevent damage to vital structures

    E   Less bone removal

5.32 **Which suture would you use when you want a resorbable suture?**

    A   Black silk suture 3–0

    B   Prolene 4–0

    C   Vicryl 3–0

    D   Vicryl Rapide 4–0

    E   Monocryl

5.30 ABCD

Damage to the inferior dental and/or lingual nerves may occur during removal of lower third molars. As these nerves are sensory this may result in anaesthesia or paraesthesia but not paralysis. Dry socket is a common complication of removal of lower molars.

5.31 ADE

Marsupialisation is a technique where the cyst cavity is opened via a window in the lining and this is sutured to the mucosa, so that the cyst cavity communicates with the oral cavity. Enucleation is a technique in which the whole cyst is removed and the cyst cavity closed to the oral cavity. Marsupialisation involves less bone removal and hence may prevent damage to adjacent vital structures. The cyst cavity is then open for inspection as it heals, but the cavity may be difficult for the patient to clean. It also has the disadvantage that only a portion of the cyst lining is available for histological analysis.

5.32 CDE

Monocryl, Vicryl and Vicryl Rapide are all types of resorbable suture.

5.33 **An incisional biopsy is indicated in the diagnosis of which of the following lesions?**

A   Squamous cell carcinoma on the lateral border of the tongue

B   Fibroepithelial polyp on the buccal mucosa

C   Capillary haemangioma on the lower lip

D   Sublingual keratosis

E   A palpable lump in the submandibular gland

5.34 **Identify the sutures labelled i–iii in the figure. Choose from the list of options below.**

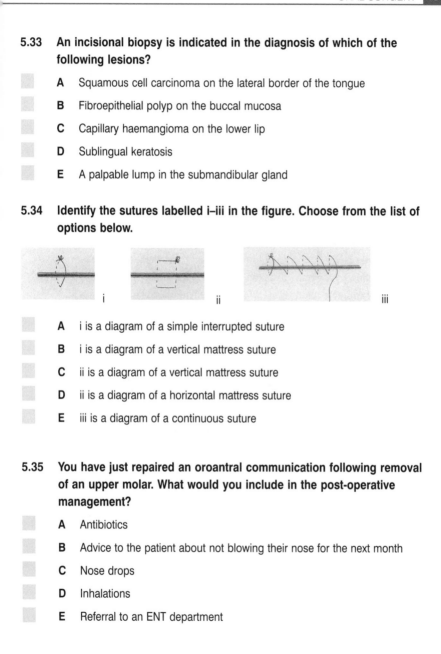

A   i is a diagram of a simple interrupted suture

B   i is a diagram of a vertical mattress suture

C   ii is a diagram of a vertical mattress suture

D   ii is a diagram of a horizontal mattress suture

E   iii is a diagram of a continuous suture

5.35 **You have just repaired an oroantral communication following removal of an upper molar. What would you include in the post-operative management?**

A   Antibiotics

B   Advice to the patient about not blowing their nose for the next month

C   Nose drops

D   Inhalations

E   Referral to an ENT department

5.33   AD

Incisional biopsies are indicated for oral squamous cell carcinomas and sublingual keratosis. A fibroepithelial polyp on the buccal mucosa should be removed in its entirety – hence an excisional biopsy is indicated. A capillary haemangioma should not have a biopsy carried out on it. A lump in the submandibular gland may be investigated by fine needle aspiration but not an open incisional biopsy.

5.34   ADE

i is a simple interrupted suture, commonly used for intra and extra oral wounds. ii is a horizontal mattress suture often used in bleeding tooth sockets. iii is a continuous suture, which has the advantage of being quicker to do than multiple interrupted sutures. However, care must be taken when tying the knots of a continuous suture because if they come undone, the whole suture line will come undone.

5.35   ACD

After the closure of an oro-antral communication a patient should be advised to avoid blowing their nose until the surgical site has healed, usually 10–14 days. Antibiotics, nose drops and inhalations are often prescribed. The repair usually heals without on-going sinus problems, so patients do not usually need to be referred to ENT.

5.36 **Which of the following could occur following a fracture of the zygoma?**

A   Anosmia

B   Bruising in the ipsilateral upper buccal sulcus

C   Anaesthesia of the ipsilateral cheek

D   Epistaxis

E   Diplopia

5.37 **Which of the following are common signs and symptoms of a fracture of the zygomatic arch?**

A   Limitation of mouth opening

B   Deviation of the mandible on opening to the ipsilateral side

C   Deviation of the mandible on opening to the contralateral side

D   Diplopia

E   Epistaxis

5.38 **Regarding operating on the submandibular gland:**

A   Damage to the lingual nerve will cause loss of sensation to the posterior third of the tongue

B   The submandibular gland wraps around the posterior border of mylohyoid

C   The buccal branch of the facial nerve is at risk of surgical trauma

D   The hypoglossal nerve is seen to loop under the submandibular duct

E   The safest site for an incision is on the lower border of the mandible to prevent damage to the facial nerve

5.36 BCDE

Signs and symptoms of a fractured zygoma include: anaesthesia or paraesthesia of the cheek, side of nose and upper lip due to damage to the infra-orbital nerve; epistaxis (nose bleed) as blood drains out of the maxillary antrum; and diplopia (double vision), usually due to oedema around the eye and bruising of the upper buccal sulcus. Anosmia or loss of smell does not usually occur.

5.37 AB

Fractured zygomatic arches frequently cause difficulty in mandibular movements due to the fractured pieces impinging on the temporalis muscle and underlying mandibular coronoid process. When patients try to open their mouth their lower jaw will deviate towards the fractured side as the mandible will not translate in the normal manner. Epistaxis or diplopia does not usually occur unless there are other associated injuries.

5.38 B

The lingual nerve supplies the anterior two-thirds of the tongue and the glossopharyngeal nerve supplies the posterior third of the tongue. Incisions are usually sited two finger widths below the lower border of the mandible to avoid damage to the marginal mandibular branch of the facial nerve, the branch at greatest risk of damage during surgery of this gland. The lingual nerve loops around the submandibular duct, not the hypoglossal nerve.

5.39 **Regarding the muscles of mastication:**

   A The temporalis can be divided into anterior, middle and posterior fibres, all of which carry out the same movements

   B The anterior and middle fibres contribute to elevation of the mandible

   C The middle and posterior fibres contribute to elevation of the mandible

   D The anterior and middle fibres contribute to retrusion of the mandible

   E The posterior fibres contribute to retrusion of the mandible

5.40 **Regarding the ligaments of the temporomandibular joint:**

   A The temporomandibular ligament is related to the lateral aspect of the joint

   B The stylomandibular ligament is a remnant of the deep cervical fascia as it passes lateral to the parotid gland

   C The stylohyoid ligament extends from the tip of the styloid process to the lingula

   D The sphenomandibular ligament extends from the spine of the sphenoid to the lingula

   E The sphenomandibular ligament is a remnant of Meckel's cartilage

5.41 **Regarding the temporomandibular joint:**

   A The articular surfaces of the joint are covered with fibrocartilage

   B The articular surfaces are covered with hyaline cartilage

   C The articular disc is composed of hyaline cartilage

   D The middle part of the disc is the vascular area

   E The disc attaches to the articular capsule anteriorly

5.39 BE

The temporalis muscle can be divided into three parts which carry out different movements. The posterior fibres retract the mandible, and the remaining fibres of the muscle elevate the mandible.

5.40 ADE

The stylomandibular ligament is a remnant of the deep cervical fascia as it passes medial to the parotid gland. The stylohyoid ligament extends from the tip of the styloid process to the angle of the mandible.

5.41 A

The articular surfaces of the temporomandibular joint are covered with fibrocartilage, and the articular disc is also made of fibrocartilage. The middle part of the disc is avascular. The disc attaches to the anterior margin of the articular eminence, the articular margin of the condyle and the lateral pterygoid muscle.

6

Child Dental Health and Orthodontics

6.1 Trauma to deciduous teeth may affect the developing permanent teeth. Which of the following are common side-effects that are seen in permanent teeth following trauma to deciduous teeth?

- **A** Altered eruption
- **B** Crown dilaceration
- **C** Dens in dente
- **D** Enamel hypoplasia
- **E** Osteoma

6.2 Which of the following statements are correct regarding the Hall technique of fitting preformed metallic crowns on teeth?

- **A** Requires extensive caries removal prior to fitting of the crown
- **B** Requires administration of local anaesthesia prior to commencing the procedure
- **C** Has equal success in the primary and secondary dentition
- **D** Is a useful technique when a child has little or no experience of invasive dental treatment
- **E** Requires occlusal reduction so as not to create a high restoration

6.3 A child has had trauma to one of their upper deciduous incisors. Which of the following would suggest that active treatment on the traumatised tooth is usually required?

- **A** The upper left A is extruded
- **B** The upper left A has been intruded with the crown pushed labially
- **C** The upper left A has been intruded with the crown pushed lingually
- **D** The upper left A has sustained a luxation injury and is interfering with the occlusion
- **E** The upper left A was avulsed 10 minutes ago and has been kept in milk by the parent

6.1   ABD

Trauma to a deciduous tooth often causes damage to the developing permanent successor. Common effects are: hypomineralisation of the enamel, crown dilaceration, crown-root dilaceration, odontome formation, arrest of root formation and sequestration or resorption of the developing tooth germ. Damaged developing permanent teeth may also show altered eruption following the trauma.

6.2   D

The Hall technique is used for primary molar teeth and does not involve administration of local anaesthesia or tooth preparation. It is useful if a child has no experience of dental treatment and is uncooperative. Despite the restoration feeling high when the crown is fitted, it tends to resolve in a few days and usually does not need adjustment.

6.3   ABD

Active treatment is required if the tooth is mobile and a danger to the airway, if it interfering with the occlusion, is extremely painful or the apex has been displaced into the underlying developing permanent tooth germ. It is not common practice to reimplant deciduous teeth as this may further damage the underlying permanent tooth germ and may introduce infection into the area.

6.4 **Which of the statements are correct regarding a 9-year-old patient?**

A   Children of this age should never be advised to use toothpaste with more than 1000 ppm

B   Fluoride tablets would be the best way of administering fluoride if the child shows evidence of caries or a high caries risk and lives in a non-fluoridated area

C   If the child lives in a fluoridated area of 1 ppm then you must advise them to use non-fluoridated toothpaste as they are at risk from fluorosis

D   Mottling of enamel can occur with systemic administration of fluoride in water at a level of 1 ppm

E   You could consider advising the use of a fluoride mouthwash if indicated by caries risk

6.5 **Which of the following may be indications for using the Hall technique (of using preformed metal crowns) to manage carious primary molars**

A   A lower second deciduous molar tooth with a Class II carious lesion and signs and symptoms of irreversible pulpitis

B   A lower second deciduous molar tooth with a Class II carious lesion that is cavitated

C   A lower second deciduous molar tooth with a non-cavitated Class I carious lesion in a child who is unable to accept a conventional restoration or a fissure sealant

D   A lower second deciduous molar tooth with a broken down crown that would be considered unrestorable with conventional techniques

E   A lower second deciduous molar tooth with a Class II carious lesion that shows radiographic signs of pulpal involvement

6.4 DE

Systemic fluoride administration has an effect on the developing dentition as well as teeth that have already erupted, and it requires a high level of compliance. At the age of 9 the crowns of the developing teeth (except the third molars) will have formed. Also at 9 years, the child should be dexterous enough to carry out oral hygiene measures. In this case regular topical administration may be the best way of administering fluoride.

Children over 6 years who are at high risk of caries can use toothpaste with 1500 ppm. Mottling can occur with any level of fluoride administration although the risks increase greatly with increasing concentration (Dean 1936).

6.5 BC

The Hall technique can be used to manage restorable deciduous molar teeth with no signs and symptoms of irreversible pulpal involvement. It is not suitable if the tooth would not be considered restorable with conventional techniques. It can be useful in uncooperative children as no tooth preparation is needed.

6.6   Regarding dento-alveolar trauma:

A   Concussion means injury to the supporting tissues of a tooth with displacement

B   Concussion means injury to the supporting tissues of a tooth without displacement

C   Luxation means displacement of a tooth

D   Subluxation means loosening of a tooth in its socket without displacement

E   Subluxation means loosening of a tooth in its socket with a dento-alveolar fracture

6.7   Which of the following could cause a crossbite?

A   Thumb-sucking habit

B   Skeletal discrepancy

C   Cleft lip and palate

D   Amelogenesis imperfecta

E   Osteogenesis imperfecta

6.8   Which of the following factors would increase a child's risk for caries?

A   Coming from an affluent family

B   Having a poorly educated mother

C   High caries rate in siblings

D   Exposure to fluoride

E   Having a decreased salivary flow rate

6.6 BCD

Luxation means displacement of a tooth. It is used to describe displacement in any direction except apically and occlusally, in which case the displacement is known as intrusion and extrusion, respectively. Concussion means that the tooth is traumatised, but it has not moved in its socket. Subluxation is used to describe loosening of a tooth without displacement, despite the fact that the word subluxation actually means partial displacement.

6.7 ABC

Anything that may alter the normal relationship of maxillary to mandibular teeth may cause a crossbite, eg a skeletal discrepancy or a cleft palate. Prolonged thumb sucking may cause tilting of the teeth and narrowing of the maxillary arch, which can also result in a crossbite.

6.8 BCE

To determine the risk status of a child for caries, socio-demographic, dental and other factors must all be considered. Children with a high risk for caries are usually in the lower socio-economic groups with poorly educated parents. The caries experience of siblings should also be taken into consideration, as a high caries experience would put the child at greater risk. Exposure to fluoride decreases the risk of caries whereas a decreased salivary flow rate increases the caries risk.

6.9   **Which of the following situations would be appropriate for using fissure sealants?**

  A   On the deciduous molars of a child with extensive caries in their deciduous teeth

  B   On the permanent molars of a child with extensive caries in their deciduous teeth

  C   In a caries-free child

  D   In a child with an impairment

  E   Only within 24 months of the eruption of the tooth in question

6.10   **Which of the following methods of topical fluoride application are appropriate in an 8-year-old child (who lives in an area with < 0.3 ppm of fluoride in the water supply)?**

  A   Toothpaste with 500 ppm of fluoride

  B   Toothpaste with 1000 ppm of fluoride

  C   0.05% fluoride mouthwash daily

  D   0.05% fluoride mouthwash weekly

  E   0.5 mg fluoride tablets daily

6.11   **The force required to bodily move a single-rooted tooth is about:**

  A   5–10 g

  B   10–50 g

  C   50–100 g

  D   100–150 g

  E   150–500 g

6.9   BD

Fissure sealants are not normally used on deciduous teeth. They are used on permanent teeth and do not need to be placed within a limited time of the tooth erupting. They should be considered for children who have extensive caries in their primary dentition, children with impairments and in children whose general health would be jeopardised by either the development of oral disease or the need for dental treatment.

6.10   BC

Mouthwashes are contra-indicated in young children, but a child of 8 years should be able to use them. The ideal is 0.05% fluoride daily, but it may be substituted by a 0.2% mouthwash once a week. A fluoride concentration of 500 ppm in toothpaste for an 8-year-old is too low, it should 1000 ppm. Fluoride 1 mg tablets are appropriate for 8-year-olds.

6.11   D

The force required to move a tooth bodily is greater than that required to tip a tooth as it is distributed over a greater area of the periodontal ligament. For a single-rooted tooth about 100–150 g force is required for bodily movement. Larger forces are required for multi-rooted teeth.

6.12 Excessive force during orthodontic treatment may result in:

A Root resorption

B Mobility of teeth

C Increase in anchorage

D Increased caries rate

E Delayed tooth movement

6.13 Advantages of removable appliance therapy include:

A They are easier to clean than fixed appliances

B Intermaxillary traction is possible

C Groups of teeth can be moved together

D Speech is rarely affected

E Bodily tooth movements are possible

6.14 Which of the following statements are true?

A Balancing extractions are removal of the same tooth (or adjacent tooth) on the same side in the opposing arch

B Balancing extractions are removal of the same tooth (or adjacent tooth) in the same arch on the other side

C Compensating extractions are removal of the same tooth (or adjacent tooth) on the same side in the opposing arch

D Compensating extractions are removal of the same tooth (or adjacent tooth) in the same arch on the other side

6.12   ABE

One of the complications of orthodontic treatment is root resorption, both lateral and apical. This occurs more frequently when greater forces are used. Teeth may also become mobile and tooth movement can be delayed rather than speeded up. Use of excessive force does not cause an increase in caries rate but may result in a decrease in anchorage.

6.13   AC

Intermaxillary traction is not possible with removable appliances. Removable appliances tip teeth rather than move them bodily. They often affect speech more than a fixed appliance as the baseplate is bulky and encroaches on the tongue space.

6.14   BC

Balancing extractions refers to extractions on the other side of the arch and compensating extractions to extractions in the opposing arch.

6.15 **Which of the following are normal cephalometric values for Caucasians?**

   A SNA: 79° ± 3°

   B Upper central incisor to maxillary plane:109° ± 6°

   C ANB: 3° ± 2°

   D MMPA: 35° ± 4°

   E MMPA: 27° ± 4°

6.16 **Which of the following landmarks are used to describe the various cephalometric planes?**

   A S to N: Frankfort plane

   B Po to Or: Frankfort plane

   C Po to Or: Mandibular plane

   D PNS to ANS: Maxillary plane

   E PNS to ANS: Mandibular plane

6.17 **Which descriptions of the following commonly used cephalometric landmarks are correct?**

   A Sella is the anterior wall of sella turcica

   B Nasion is the most anterior point on the fronto-nasal suture

   C Orbitale is the most superior point on the orbital rim

   D Porion is the most anterior point on the mandibular symphysis

   E Menton is the most inferior point on the mandibular symphysis

6.15   BCE

Normal values are as follows:

- SNA: 81° ± 3°
- SNB: 79° ± 3°
- MMPA: 27° ± 4°

6.16   BD

Go to Me: Mandibular plane.

6.17   BE

Sella is the central point of the sella turcica, and orbitale is the most inferior point on the orbital rim. The pogonion is the most anterior point on the mandibular symphysis, whereas porion is the uppermost anterior point on the external auditory meatus.

6.18 A 14-year-old boy arrives at your surgery with an absent upper right permanent canine. The upper left permanent canine erupted 12 months ago. Which of the following observations would suggest that the upper right canine was buccally impacted?

   A A palpable bulge in the anterior palate on the right

   B A proclined permanent upper right lateral incisor

   C A buccally situated upper canine on the other side

   D A retroclined permanent upper right lateral incisor

   E A buccal bulge in the alveolus in the region of the canine on the right hand side

6.19 A 13-year-old girl attends your dental practice. She is a thumb sucker. What type of malocclusion would she be likely to have?

   A Anterior openbite

   B Posterior openbite

   C Posterior crossbite

   D Increased overbite

   E Decreased overbite

6.20 A 15-year-old girl attends your surgery with a midline diastema. Which of the following could possibly be a cause of a midline diastema?

   A Normal development

   B Midline conical supernumerary

   C Hypodontia

   D Prominent lingual fraenum

   E Microdontia

6.18 BE

The majority of impacted canines are palatal and unilateral. A proclined lateral incisor may indicate the unerupted canine is buccal, as the unerupted tooth pushes the root tip of the lateral incisor palatally and its crown buccally. A palpable bulge buccally may also indicate that the tooth is lying buccally. A buccally impacted or erupted canine on one side has no bearing on the other as impactions are not symmetrical.

6.19 ACE

Thumb sucking usually leads to proclination of the upper incisors and retroclination of the lower incisors which can cause a decreased overbite or an anterior open bite. A posterior crossbite often occurs due to over-activity of the buccinator muscles.

6.20 BCE

Diastemas due to normal development (physiological spacing) are likely to close spontaneously with eruption of the permanent canine (11–13 years). A prominent lingual fraenum will have no bearing on the position of the upper incisors.

6.21 **Regarding pulp treatment of primary teeth:**

   A   Pulpotomy means the removal of the entire coronal and radicular pulp

   B   Beechwood creosote is used for one-visit pulpotomies on vital pulps

   C   Formocresol is used for vital pulpotomies

   D   15.5% ferric sulphate can be used instead of beechwood creosote

   E   Cvek's pulpotomy is done for vital pulps

6.22 **Which of the following factors make restoring deciduous teeth different from restoring permanent teeth?**

   A   Crowns of deciduous teeth are more bulbous than permanent teeth

   B   Crowns of permanent teeth are more bulbous than deciduous teeth

   C   The enamel is laid down in a more orderly fashion in deciduous teeth

   D   Deciduous teeth have broader contact points than permanent teeth

   E   Deciduous teeth have narrower contact points than permanent teeth

6.23 **Which of the following types of behaviour management techniques are used when treating children in the dental surgery?**

   A   Tell, show, do

   B   Modelling

   C   Sensitisation

   D   Positive reinforcement

   E   Behaviour shaping

6.21 C

Pulpectomy means the removal of the entire coronal and radicular pulp. Beechwood creosote is used for devitalising pulpotomies. Formoscresol is used for vital pulpotomies, and 15.5% ferric sulphate can be used instead. Cvek's pulpotomy is carried out on permanent teeth, usually incisors, in an effort to allow apex formation to occur following trauma to the pulp.

6.22 AD

The crowns of deciduous teeth are more bulbous than permanent teeth and their contact points are wider. The enamel on deciduous teeth is thinner. The enamel is laid down in a more orderly fashion in permanent teeth, hence they do not need to be etched for as long as deciduous teeth.

6.23 ABDE

Desensitisation, not sensitisation, is a behaviour management method used for children with pre-existing fears.

6.24   Regarding eruption dates:

A   Deciduous maxillary upper central incisors erupt at about 7 months

B   Deciduous mandibular canines erupt at about 12–16 months

C   Deciduous mandibular second molars erupt at about 21–30 months

D   Deciduous maxillary second molars erupt at about 30–34 months

E   Permanent maxillary first premolars erupt at about 10–11 years

6.25   Which of the following statements are correct?

A   The crowns of the permanent maxillary central incisors start to calcify at 3–4 months in utero

B   The permanent maxillary central incisors erupt at about age 7–8 years and the root formation is complete at about age 10

C   The crowns of the permanent maxillary canines start to calcify at birth

D   The permanent mandibular second molars erupt at about age 12–13 and root formation is complete at about age 14–15

E   The crowns of the maxillary first premolars start to form at about 18–24 months

6.26   Which of the following may be signs that a patient is not wearing their removable orthodontic appliance?

A   Difficulty inserting the appliance

B   Poor speech

C   Springs very loose at next visit

D   No evidence of wear on the appliance

E   Poor fit

6.24 ACE

Deciduous mandibular canines erupt at about 16–20 months. Deciduous mandibular and maxillary second molars erupt at about 21–30 months.

6.25 BDE

The crowns of the permanent maxillary central incisors start to calcify at 3–4 months after birth. The crowns of the permanent maxillary canines start to calcify at about age 4–5 months.

6.26 ABDE

All are signs that a patient is not wearing their appliance except that springs are usually active if the appliance has not been used.

6.27 A mother telephones your dental practice. Her 10-year-old daughter has a knocked-out upper central incisor following a roller skating accident. The mother is not sure how to re-implant the tooth, so you advise her to attend the practice with the daughter and tooth. Which of the following storage media are suitable for the avulsed tooth?

 A Milk

 B Chlorhexidine mouthwash

 C Placing the tooth in the buccal sulcus of the daughter's mouth

 D Saline or contact lens solution

 E Cold water

6.28 The following are often seen in children with non-accidental injuries:

 A Bruises of differing ages present at the same time

 B Injuries that appear consistent with the explanation of how they occurred

 C Fraenal tears

 D Injuries in the head and neck region

 E Older children are often involved

6.27 ACD

Ideally the tooth should be re-implanted as soon as possible, but if no-one on site is capable of doing it then they should bring the tooth to the surgery for re-implantation. The ideal storage medium should be as physiological as possible. Hence the tooth should not be placed in chlorhexidine mouthwash. Cold water is not ideal as it is hypotonic and may result in lysis of the periodontal ligament cells.

6.28 ACD

Non-accidental injuries occur in the head and neck region in 50% of cases. Patients often have bruises of differing ages and often present late for treatment. Injuries often appear inconsistent with the explanation of how they occurred. Injuries are often inflicted on younger rather than older children.

7

Therapeutics

7.1   **Which of the following statements about interactions with ibuprofen are correct?**

   A   Corticosteroids and ibuprofen both cause peptic ulceration and combined use should be avoided

   B   Ibuprofen can antagonise the hypotensive effects of angiotensin-converting enzyme (ACE) inhibitors (eg captopril)

   C   Ibuprofen may increase the renal clearance of digoxin, causing a decrease in plasma concentration

   D   Ibuprofen may enhance the effect of anticoagulants such as warfarin

   E   Ibuprofen increases the excretion of methotrexate

7.2   **Benzodiazepines are used for dental sedation. Which of the following are effects of benzodiazepines?**

   A   Analgesia

   B   Amnesia

   C   Anticonvulsant

   D   Antipyretic

   E   Anxiolysis

7.3   **Which of the following are undesirable effects of benzodiazepine sedative drugs?**

   A   Cardiac excitability

   B   Dreams including sexual fantasies

   C   Hypertension

   D   Paradoxical excitation, especially in teenagers

   E   Respiratory depression

7.1 ABD

Corticosteroids and ibuprofen both cause peptic ulceration and their combined use should be avoided. Ibuprofen may enhance the effect of anticoagulants such as warfarin and heparin, and can increase the risk of gastric bleeding in patients on anti-platelet drugs. Ibuprofen may decrease the renal clearance of digoxin causing an increase in plasma concentration. Ibuprofen reduces the excretion of methotrexate, which can lead to methotrexate toxicity.

7.2 BCE

Benzodiazepines have the following effects – muscle relaxation, hypnosis, sedation, anxiolysis and amnesia. They do not have analgesic or antipyretic properties.

7.3 BDE

Benzodiazepines are anxiolytic and hypnotic drugs that are thought to have their effect through benzodiazepine receptors that are associated with gamma-aminobutyric acid (GABA) receptors. They cause minimal cardiac depression and hypotension, which may well occur due to their anxiolytic effect and muscle relaxation. They also cause sexual fantasies and a degree of anterograde amnesia and occasionally cause paradoxical excitation.

7.4 **A fit and healthy 24-year-old patient has the prodromal symptoms of a cold sore on their lower lip. What could you prescribe for them?**

   A   Adcortyl in Orabase

   B   Aciclovir cream

   C   Fusidic acid cream

   D   Miconazole gel

   E   Penciclovir cream

7.5 **Which of the following drugs are known to interact in the manner described?**

   A   When taken together erythromycin causes an increase in the plasma levels of simvastatin

   B   When taken together erythromycin causes an increase in the plasma concentrations of warfarin

   C   When taken together metronidazole causes an increase in the plasma concentrations of warfarin

   D   Erythromycin causes an increase in acetaldehyde levels when taken with alcohol which may cause headache, nausea and palpitations, and so alcohol should be avoided with these antibiotics

   E   Metronidazole causes an increase in acetaldehyde levels when taken with alcohol which may cause headache, nausea and palpitations, and so alcohol should be avoided with these antibiotics

7.4 BE

Cold sores are caused by reactivation of the herpes simplex virus. Any treatment given should be antiviral and given in the prodromal phase to be most effective. Systemic therapy is not indicated in fit and healthy patients. Hence penciclovir and aciclovir are acceptable. Fusidic acid cream is antibacterial and effective against staphylococci, and it can be used in angular cheilitis. Miconazole gel is antifungal (although it does have some antibacterial effect when used for angular cheilitis). Adcortyl in Orabase is a topical steroid preparation.

7.5 ABCE

Erythromycin interacts with simvastatin and warfarin by inhibition of a cytochrome enzyme in the liver responsible for drug metabolism, resulting in an increase in plasma concentrations. Metronidazole interacts with warfarin by the same mechanism. When consumed together metronidazole blocks the enzyme acetaldehyde dehydrogenase, which is responsible for converting acetaldehyde to acetic acid and so causes an increase in level of acetaldehyde which can cause palpitations, nausea and headache. Erythromycin does not cause this inhibition.

7.6 Which of the following are known to interact in the manner described?

A The efficacy of the contraceptive pill may be reduced when a course of antibiotics is taken because the antibiotics alter the gut flora, which stops the contraceptive pill from being absorbed

B The efficacy of the contraceptive pill may be reduced when a course of antibiotics is taken because the antibiotic combine with the contraceptive drug in the gut and altering its absorption

C Tetracyclines form chelates with certain ions including Ca^{2+} and so should not be taken with foodstuffs containing milk or diary products

D Phenoxymethyl penicillin is deactivated by the low pH of the stomach and so must be given by injection

E Benzylpenicillin is deactivated by the low pH of the stomach and so must be given by injection

7.7 What is the correct mechanism of action of the following drugs?

A Amoxycillin acts by blocking cross-linking of the bacterial cell wall

B Metronidazole inhibits nucleic acid synthesis

C Clindamycin acts by blocking cross-linking of the bacterial cell wall

D Doxycycline inhibits protein synthesis by binding to bacterial ribosomes

E Clindamycin inhibits protein synthesis by binding to bacterial ribosomes

7.8 Which of the following statements are correct?

A Flumazenil is a benzodiazepine agonist

B Flumazenil is a benzodiazepine antagonist

C Benzodiazepines are commonly used anxiolytic drugs

D Benzodiazepines may be used in the treatment of epilepsy

E Carbamazepine is a benzodiazepine

7.6   CE

Antibiotics used in dentistry do alter the gut flora, and may have an effect on the efficacy of the contraceptive pill. However this is due to the combined contraceptive pill undergoing enterohepatic recycling whereby a conjugate of oestrogen and glucuronic acid that was previously excreted into the gut is hydrolysed by colonic bacteria – this releases the oestrogen, which is reabsorbed and then suppresses ovulation.

Tetracyclines form chelates with certain ions such as Ca^{2+}, Mg^{2+}, Fe^{2+} and Zn^{2+} and so should not be taken with foodstuffs containing milk or diary products, or antacids that contain calcium and magnesium salts. When prescribing tetracyclines it is advisable to tell patients to take the drug on an empty stomach or at least 60 minutes after food.

7.7   ABDE

Penicillins inhibit bacterial cell wall synthesis by blocking cross-linking. All β-lactam antibiotics have a similar mode of action. Macrolides (eg erythromycin), lincosamides (eg clindamycin) and doxycycline inhibit bacterial synthesis by binding to bacterial ribosomes.

7.8   BCD

Benzodiazepines are central nervous system depressants and act as sedatives, hypnotics, anxiolytics and anti-convulsants. Flumazenil is a benzodiazepine antagonist, commonly used to reverse the action of midazolam. Although having a name that sounds similar to benzodiazepine, carbamazepine is not a benzodiazepine.

7.9   Which of the following statements are correct?

    A   Lidocaine 0.2% with 1:80 000 adrenaline (epinephrine) is a commonly used dental local anaesthetic

    B   Lidocaine has a longer lasting anaesthetic effect than bupivacaine

    C   Plain lidocaine provides more pronounced dental anaesthesia than lidocaine with adrenaline (epinephrine)

    D   Prilocaine 3% with 0.03 IU/ml felypressin is a commonly used dental local anaesthetic

    E   Lidocaine must be stored at 4 °C

7.10   Which of the following statements are correct?

    A   A 2.2 ml cartridge of 2% lidocaine and 1:80 000 adrenaline (epinephrine) contains 4.4 mg of lidocaine

    B   Lidocaine and prilocaine contain an ester group

    C   Esters are less likely to cause allergic reactions than amides

    D   Amide local anaesthetics are metabolised by the liver

    E   Prilocaine has a much higher toxicity than lidocaine

7.11   Which of the following drugs interact with warfarin and may increase a patient's international normalised ratio (INR)?

    A   Fluconazole

    B   Vitamin K

    C   Metronidazole

    D   Erythromycin

    E   Oral contraceptives

7.9   D

Lidocaine 2% with 1:80 000 adrenaline (epinephrine) is a commonly used dental local anaesthetic. It has a more pronounced effect than lidocaine alone as adrenaline (epinephrine) causes vasoconstriction, which prevents the solution dispersing away from the site of action. Bupivacaine is a longer lasting local anaesthetic than lidocaine.

7.10   D

A 2% solution will contain 20 mg/ml, so a 2.2 ml cartridge contains 44 mg of lidocaine. Lidocaine and prilocaine contain an amide group, and as such are less likely to cause an allergic reaction than an ester-containing local anaesthetic. Lidocaine has higher toxicity than prilocaine.

7.11   ACD

Fluconazole, erythromycin and metronidazole may interact with warfarin and potentiate its action. The oral contraceptive pill and vitamin K may interact with warfarin, but they reduce its effect hence lowering the INR.

7.12 Non-steroidal anti-inflammatory drugs (NSAIDs) are best avoided in:

A Patients with a history of gastric bleeding

B Asthmatic patients

C Patients who are hypersensitive to aspirin

D Children under the age of 6 years due to the possibility of Reye's syndrome

E Patients on paracetamol

7.13 Penicillins:

A Are the antibiotic of choice for anaerobic infections

B Interfere with bacterial cell wall synthesis

C Are bacteriocidal

D Are antagonistic to tetracycline

E Rarely cause allergic reactions

7.14 What are the appropriate drugs and dosages for use in the following emergencies?

A In suspected anaphylaxis – 1:1000 adrenaline (epinephrine) 0.5 ml intravenously

B In suspected anaphylaxis – chlorphenamine 10 mg in 1 ml intramuscularly

C In a suspected angina attack – glyceryl trinitrate intramuscularly

D In a suspected diabetic hypoglycaemic collapse where the patient is unconscious – glucagon 10 mg intramuscularly

E In a suspected diabetic hypoglycaemic collapse where the patient is unconscious – 50 ml of 20% glucose intravenously

7.12 ABCD

NSAIDs should be avoided in any patient with a history of hypersensitivity to aspirin or any other NSAID. They should also be avoided in patients with gastric/duodenal ulceration, and if it is necessary to prescribe them, then they should be given in conjunction with a selective inhibitor of cyclo-oxygenase–2 or gastroprotective treatment. Reye's syndrome can be caused by patients under the age of 16 years taking aspirin and hence it should be avoided in children. Patients on paracetamol can take NSAIDs as well as they have different modes of action and do not interact.

7.13 BCD

The penicillins all act by interfering with bacterial cell wall synthesis, by inhibiting cross-linking of the mucopeptides in the cell wall and as such are bacteriocidal. Bacteria are attacked when cells are dividing and so in theory antibiotics that are bacteriostatic would decrease the efficacy of bacteriocidal drugs. However, this doesn't often cause a problem but tetracycline and penicillin are antagonistic and should not be used at the same time. Metronidazole is the antibiotic of choice for anaerobic infections.

7.14 BE

In suspected anaphylaxis 0.5 ml of 1:1000 adrenaline (epinephrine) is given intramuscularly as is chlorphenamine 10 mg in 1 ml (also intramuscularly). In an angina attack glyceryl trinitrate is usually administered sublingually. In a hypoglycaemic collapse glucagon 1 mg is given intramuscularly and/or 50 ml of 20% glucose intravenously.

7.15 Paracetamol is:

  A Anti-pyretic

  B Anti-inflammatory

  C Locally acting

  D Hepatotoxic in overdose

  E Taken in doses of 500 mg –1 g four times a day

7.16 Which of the following drugs and doses are commonly used in the treatment of atypical facial pain?

  A Amitriptyline 10–25 mg daily

  B Nortriptyline 10–25 mg daily

  C Protirelin 10–25 mg daily

  D Fluoxetine 20 mg daily

  E Flumazenil 20 mg daily

7.17 Which of the following are anti-fungal drugs?

  A Miconazole

  B Aciclovir

  C Chlorhexidine

  D Nystatin

  E Itraconazole

7.15 ADE

Paracetamol is a centrally acting analgesic with anti-pyretic properties. Unlike the NSAIDs it does not have anti-inflammatory properties. It is hepatotoxic in high doses.

7.16 ABD

Amitriptyline and nortriptyline are both tricyclic antidepressants and are used in the treatment of atypical facial pain. Fluoxetine is a selective serotonin reuptake inhibitor and also used in the treatment of facial pain. Protirelin is a hypothalamic-releasing hormone which stimulates the release of thyrotrophin from the pituitary gland and so is not used for treatment of atypical facial pain. Flumazenil is a benzodiazepine antagonist used to reverse the central sedative effects of benzodiazepines.

7.17 ADE

Miconazole is an imidazole anti-fungal drug, Nystatin is a polyene anti-fungal drug and itraconazole is a triazole anti-fungal. Aciclovir is an anti-viral drug and chlorhexidine is an antiseptic.

7.18   Which of the following must always be included in a prescription?

A   The name and address of the prescriber

B   The age of the patient

C   The date of prescription

D   The dose of the drug in numbers and words

E   The address of the patient

7.19   Which of the following drug doses and concentrations are correct for using in an anaphylactic reaction?

A   Adrenaline (epinephrine) 0.5 ml of 1:100 intramuscularly

B   Adrenaline (epinephrine) 0.5 ml of 1:1000 intramuscularly

C   Hydrocortisone sodium succinate 2 mg intravenously

D   Hydrocortisone sodium succinate 20 mg intravenously

E   Hydrocortisone sodium succinate 200 mg intravenously

7.20   Which of the following drugs cause lichenoid reaction?

A   β-Blockers

B   Nifedipine

C   Allopurinol

D   Phenytoin

E   Anti-malarials

7.18 ACE

The name and address of the prescriber, the date of prescription and the address of the patient must be included. It is desirable to include the age and date of birth of the patient, but this is a legal requirement for only prescription-only medicines for patients under 12 years of age. The drug dose only needs to be put in words and figures if it is a controlled drug.

7.19 BE

Appropriate treatment of a suspected anaphylactic attack involves 0.5–1 ml of a 1:1000 solution of adrenaline (epinephrine) administered intramuscularly. Hydrocortisone sodium succinate 200 mg intravenously should also be given.

7.20 ACE

β-Blockers, anti-malarials and allopurinol cause lichenoid reactions. Phenytoin and nifedipine cause gingival hyperplasia.

7.21   **Which of the following drugs cause a dry mouth?**

A   Heavy metal poisoning

B   Atropine

C   Tricyclic antidepressants

D   Anti-emetics

E   Anti-malarials

7.22   **You have prescribed oral metronidazole. What instructions do you need to give the patient?**

A   Take the tablets twice a day

B   Take the tablets three times a day

C   Take the tablets until the pain has subsided

D   Avoid drinking alcohol while taking the tablets

E   Take the whole course as prescribed

7.23   **Which of the following are correct regarding the action of local anaesthetic agents?**

A   Local anaesthetics block hydrogen channels

B   Local anaesthetics block sodium channels

C   Local anaesthetics block potassium channels

D   Local anaesthetics have membrane-stabilising properties

E   Local anaesthetics have membrane-activating properties

7.21 BCD

Anti-malarials cause lichenoid reactions. Atropine is an anti-muscarinic drug (formerly known as anti-cholinergics). It reduces gastric and salivary secretions, and hence causes a dry mouth. Some tricyclics and anti-emetics also cause dry mouth.

7.22 BDE

Oral metronidazole is usually prescribed as 200 mg or 400 mg tablets taken three times a day. It is important that patients do not drink alcohol while taking metronidazole as the two will interact. Antibiotic courses should be completed as prescribed and not stopped when pain subsides.

7.23 BD

Local anaesthetics work by producing reversible inhibition of impulses in peripheral nerves by virtue of their membrane-stabilising properties. They act by blocking sodium channels and preventing membrane depolarisation.

7.24   Aspirin:

   A   Is an NSAID

   B   Prevents the synthesis of prostaglandin E_3

   C   Is anti-pyretic

   D   May cause gastric mucosal irritation and bleeding

   E   Is commonly used as an analgesic for children

7.25   Patients on oral anticoagulants:

   A   Carry a blue warning card

   B   Must wear a MedicAlert bracelet

   C   Have their anti-coagulation monitored by regular blood tests to measure their INR

   D   Have a target therapeutic range of INR 2–3

   E   Must stop their anticoagulants 3 days prior to tooth extractions

7.26   Which of the following drugs can be safely prescribed in pregnancy?

   A   Metronidazole

   B   Paracetamol

   C   Prilocaine

   D   Miconazole

   E   Amoxycillin

7.24 ACD

Aspirin is an NSAID which acts by preventing the synthesis of prostaglandin E_2. It is anti-pyretic by virtue of its action on the hypothalamus and inhibition of prostaglandin synthesis, which is a mediator of febrile response to infections. It should not be used for children as it can cause Reye's syndrome.

7.25 C

Blue warning cards are steroid cards. MedicAlert bracelets are not necessarily worn by patients on warfarin, although some may wear them depending on their medical history. Patients on anticoagulants have a target range that their INR is meant to stay between. This will vary depending on the condition for which they are taking the anticoagulants, for example the therapeutic range for prophylaxis of deep vein thrombosis is 2–2.5 and the therapeutic range for patients with prosthetic heart valves is 3.5. Depending on a patient's INR it may not be necessary to stop their anticoagulants prior to extractions, as many extractions can be carried out safely without altering the warfarin dose.

7.26 BE

Care must always be taken when prescribing drugs during pregnancy. Metronidazole, prilocaine and miconazole should be avoided as far as possible.

7.27 **Which of the following drugs commonly cause gingival hyperplasia?**

   A   Nifedipine

   B   Phenytoin

   C   Ciclosporin

   D   Diltiazem

   E   Carbamazepine

7.28 **Which of the following are well known side effects of the named drugs?**

   A   Nifedipine may cause gingival hyperplasia

   B   Gentamicin may cause 'red man syndrome'

   C   Carbamazepine may cause a skin rash

   D   Clindamycin may cause pseudomembranous colitis

   E   Aspirin may cause Reye's syndrome

7.29 **Which of the following are complications of long-term steroid therapy?**

   A   Striae

   B   Hypotension

   C   Adrenal suppression

   D   Osteoporosis

   E   Weight loss

7.27 ABCD

Carbamazepine causes erythema multiforme, whereas the others may cause gingival hyperplasia.

7.28 ACDE

Vancomycin causes 'red man syndrome'.

7.29 ACD

Long-term steroid therapy has many complications including striae on the skin, hypertension, adrenal suppression, osteoporosis and weight gain.

7.30 **Which of the following may be signs and symptoms of lidocaine overdose:**

   A   Light headedness

   B   Tachycardia

   C   Convulsions

   D   Hypertension

   E   Hyperventilation

7.31 **Erythromycin:**

   A   Is a macrolide drug

   B   Is active against some penicillinase resistant staphylococci

   C   Is active against *Chlamydia* and mycoplasmas

   D   Should not be used during pregnancy

   E   Is given to an adult in a regimen of 250–500 mg three times daily for 5 days

7.32 **Tetracyclines:**

   A   Are broad-spectrum antibiotics

   B   Are absorbed better when taken with milk

   C   May be used as a mouthwash in a dose of 25 mg dissolved in a little water and held in the mouth

   D   Cause intrinsic staining of teeth

   E   Cause extrinsic staining of teeth

7.30 AC

Signs and symptoms of lidocaine overdose include light headedness, confusion, twitching leading to convulsions, hypotension, bradycardia and depression of respiration.

7.31 ABC

Erythromycin is a macrolide-type drug. It is safe to use in pregnancy and is prescribed in a regimen of 250–500 mg four times daily for 5 days. It is active against some penicillinase resistant staphylococci, although many are now becoming resistant to it.

7.32 AD

Tetracyclines are broad-spectrum antibiotics which bind to calcium and hence get deposited in teeth and bones. They cause intrinsic staining of teeth if taken during tooth development, and as such should not be prescribed to pregnant women and to children up to 12 years of age. Their absorption is decreased when taken with milk. Tetracycline mouthwash is used to reduce secondary infection when patients have oral ulceration. A 250 mg capsule is broken and dissolved in a little water and used as a mouthwash three times daily.

8

Dental
Materials

8.1 **Which of the following statements are correct regarding alginate impression materials?**

A The setting time is controlled by the amount of potassium sulphate

B Phenylalanine may be added to provide a disinfection action

C Some alginates can be stored for up to 5 days in 100% relative humidity before significant dimensional changes occur

D The best way to delay the setting is by using a thinner mix

E Soaking the impression for 10 minutes in 0.5% hypochlorite is more effective than spraying with the same solution

8.2 **Which of the following statements regarding composite bonding agents are correct?**

A Bonding agents are used to provide an adequate bond with dentine

B Bonding agents provide a micromechanical bond to dentine

C Bonding agents bond to enamel via a hybrid layer

D Most bonding agents are more effective when used with dry tooth surfaces than moist surfaces

E The need for a protective liner is eliminated with the use of bonding agents

8.3 **Which of the following statements are correct?**

A Bleaching systems can adversely affect microfilled composites

B Hypochlorite is a type of denture cleanser

C Alkaline perborate is a type of denture cleanser

D Organic solvents can be used as a denture cleanser

E Fissure sealants all contain fluoride to aid remineralisation of existing incipient lesions

8.1 C

The setting time is controlled by the amount of sodium phosphate, which is a retarder. Quaternary ammonium compounds or chlorhexidine provide self-disinfection. Alginates should be poured promptly because of dimensional changes when stored in air and water. The best way to delay the setting is to reduce the temperature of the water and not the consistency of the mix which results in lower tear strength. A 10-minute soak in 0.5% hypochlorite and a 10-minute wait after spraying with the same solution are both effective for inactivating viruses.

8.2 AB

Bonding agents are used with composite to provide an adequate bond with both enamel and dentine. Bonding with etched enamel is micromechanical in nature. Bonding with dentine is via removal of the smear layer, formation of a hybrid layer by the penetration of the bonding agent in the exposed collagen, which provides micromechanical retention to dentine. Most bonding agents bond more effectively with moist tooth surfaces, rather than dry or very wet surfaces. The use of a protective liner is recommended for deep cavities.

8.3 BC

Bleaching agents do not adversely affect gold alloy, amalgam, microfilled composites or porcelain but can roughen some microhybrid composites. Organic solvents, eg chloroform, should not be used as a denture cleanser as they can dissolve or craze acrylic dentures. Fissure sealants may be based on glass ionomer that releases fluoride, which may remineralise an existing incipient lesion. Those based on unfilled composite resin do not promote remineralisation but prevent further demineralisation.

8.4 **Which of the following statements are true regarding denture soft liners?**

A Soft liners can only be used for a few weeks

B Soft liners can all be processed at the chair side

C Soft liners may become harder over time due to leaching out of aromatic esters

D Silicone-based liners are particularly prone to hardening over time

E Fungal growth may occur on soft liners and present as hard raised spots

8.5 **Which of the following statements are true of glass ionomers?**

A Glass ionomers set as a result of metallic bridges between the Al^{3+} and the fluoride ions

B The set of the material is slow and may take 24 hours so it is advisable to protect it with unfilled resin or varnish

C Etching of dentine and enamel is advised to aid retention

D Cavities with less than 1 mm of dentine should have a calcium hydroxide liner in place

E The fluoride in glass ionomer is released over a period of 2 years

8.6 **Which of the following statements regarding flowable resin composites are correct?**

A Flowable resin composites have lower amounts of filler than conventional composites

B Flowable resin composites show a higher modulus of elasticity than conventional resin composites

C Flowable resin composites allow for better adaptation of material to the angles and corners of a cavity preparation

D Flowable resin composites are less able to bear stress compared with conventional resin composites, and are not indicated in areas where a high mechanical load will be anticipated

E Flowable resin composites are hydrophilic and hence good moisture control with rubber dam is not necessary

8.4 CE

Soft liners can be divided into short-term (days) or long-term liners (which can last for months). The methacrylate-based liners may be either heat or chemically cured. The former is processed in the laboratory while the latter can be chair side or laboratory based. Methacrylate-based liners often consist of poly (methyl/ethyl/ methacrylate) copolymers with a plasticiser, which may be an aromatic ester with or without alcohol. If the plasticiser leaches out the hardness of the liner is affected. Silicone-based polymers do not harden with time as they do not contain plasticisers. Silicone liners may support the growth of candidal species.

8.5 BCDE

Glass ionomers set as a result of metallic bridges between the Al^{3+} and Ca^{2+} ions. Glass ionomer may be used without cavity preparation, with etching of dentine and enamel. The fluoride in glass ionomer is released over a period of 2 years; a high concentration is released soon after placement but this reduces to a constant lower level within one week for most materials.

8.6 ACD

Flowable resin composites are hydrophobic like all resin composite materials and good moisture control is critical in their placement, and hence the use of rubber dam is advisable. Flowable resin composites have a lower modulus of elasticity (flexibility) than conventional resin composites which may have a bearing in reducing stresses that may arise due to polymerisation shrinkage.

8.7 **Which of the following statements are correct?**

A   Thermal diffusivity is the ability of a material to conduct heat

B   Wear is abrasion (with or without a chemical) of a substance

C   Resilience is a measure of how hard it is to bend a material

D   Creep is the slow dimensional change under load

E   Stress is the internal force per unit cross-sectional area acting on a material

8.8 **Regarding dental amalgam:**

A   It is a mixture of silver alloy and mercury

B   It can be composed of spherical particles, irregular particles or a mixture of the two

C   Gamma–2 is the name given to the silver–mercury product formed during amalgamation

D   Dimensional change is said to be negative if an amalgam expands during setting

E   Titration is the process of mixing the silver alloy and mercury

8.9 **The advantages of using a high-copper amalgam over a low-copper amalgam are:**

A   High copper amalgam has more gamma–2 phase and is therefore stronger than low copper amalgam

B   High copper amalgam has less gamma–2 phase and is therefore stronger than low copper amalgam

C   High copper amalgams show less corrosion than low copper amalgams

D   High copper levels prevent amalgams from expanding when contaminated with saliva

8.7 BDE

Thermal diffusivity is the rate at which temperature changes spread through materials, thermal conductivity is the ability of a material to conduct heat. Resilience is the energy absorbed by a material undergoing elastic deformation (up to its elastic limit) whereas stiffness is a measure of how hard it is to bend a material.

8.8 AB

Dental amalgam is a mixture of silver alloy and mercury. Gamma–1 is the name given to silver–mercury alloy, gamma is the name given to the silver alloy and the tin–mercury product is called gamma-2. Dimensional change is said to be negative if an amalgam contracts during setting. The process of mixing amalgam is called trituration.

8.9 BC

High-copper amalgam has almost no gamma–2 phase and is therefore stronger than low-copper amalgam, and shows less corrosion. It is the zinc in amalgam that was previously responsible for their high expansion rate when contaminated with saliva. Zinc has now been virtually eliminated from modern dental amalgams.

8.10 Regarding glass ionomers:

A   The powder is an aluminosilicate glass

B   They are mixed by adding the powder to the liquid incrementally

C   They release fluoride

D   Following initial placement they should be protected from dehydration

E   They have no effect on the pulp

8.11 Regarding compomers:

A   They release substantially more fluoride than glass ionomers

B   Their wear resistance is less than resin composites

C   They are more soluble than glass ionomers

D   They are stronger than glass ionomers

E   They bond to both enamel and dentine

8.12 With regard to cermets:

A   They are metal reinforced glass ionomer cermets

B   They are radiopaque

C   They show less wear resistance than conventional glass ionomers

D   They release more fluoride than conventional glass ionomers

E   They are used in areas where aesthetics is not a primary consideration

8.10   ACD

Glass ionomers are based on polyacrylic acid and should be mixed by adding all the powder to the liquid in one go. They do release fluoride. Following initial setting they are sensitive to dehydration and must be protected otherwise crazing or surface cracks will appear. They cause a slight inflammatory reaction in the pulp which usually resolves in a few weeks.

8.11   BD

Compomers release about a tenth of the fluoride released by glass ionomers and are less soluble than glass ionomers. They do not bond to enamel and dentine, so an intermediate bonding system is needed.

8.12   ABE

Cermets as the name suggests are ceramic metal glass, they contain either silver or gold as the metal. They are radiopaque and show better wear resistance than glass ionomers, but release less fluoride. They are aesthetically poor and hence used when aesthetics is not the primary consideration.

8.13 Regarding zinc phosphate cements:

A The powder is primarily zinc phosphate and the liquid a solution of phosphoric acid

B They have an endothermic setting reaction

C They are acidic initially, but then the pH increases to nearly neutral in 48 hours

D Retention is via chemical bonding

E The cement is mixed on a waxed paper mixing pad

8.14 Regarding zinc oxide–eugenol cements:

A Eugenol is obtundent to the pulp

B The setting reaction of zinc oxide–eugenol is retarded by water

C Eugenol inhibits free radical polymerisation

D Zinc oxide–eugenol cements may be used as a base or a temporary luting material

E When mixing, all the powder is added to the liquid in one go

8.15 Regarding alginate impression materials:

A Alginate impression material contains sodium phosphate to act as an accelerator

B The set alginate impression is a hydrocolloid gel

C It contains large quantities of water, which will evaporate and cause the impression to shrink and change shape

D If the impression is stored in water it will absorb water and expand

E The strength and flexibility of an alginate impression is increased if a thinner mixture (ie more water to powder) is used.

8.13 AC

Zinc phosphate cements have an exothermic setting reaction, which is why they are mixed on a cooled glass slab and not a waxed paper mixing pad. Their retention is via mechanical interlocking rather than chemical bonding.

8.14 ACD

Eugenol is a phenol derivative that can reduce pulpal irritation and has some anti-bacterial properties. Zinc oxide–eugenol cements can be used as either a base or a temporary luting cement depending on the thickness of the material. The setting reaction of zinc oxide–eugenol is accelerated by water and hence the material sets faster in the mouth than outside the mouth. Eugenol does inhibit free radical polymerisation and so may delay the setting of dental composites. When mixing the material the powder is added incrementally to the liquid.

8.15 BCD

Alginate impression materials contain sodium phosphate as a retarder. The sodium phosphate reacts with soluble calcium ions, and after all the sodium phosphate has reacted, the sodium alginate reacts with the calcium ions and calcium alginate is formed (which is a gel). The thicker the mixture of alginate (that is the greater the amount of powder to water) the less flexible and stronger the impression material will be.

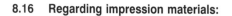

8.16 Regarding impression materials:

A Polysulphide elastomeric impression materials have higher tear resistance than alginate

B Condensation cured silicones impression materials have shorter setting times than polysulphide elastomeric impression materials

C Polyether impression materials absorb water under conditions of humidity as they are hydrophilic

D The tear resistance of polysulphide impression materials is worse than the tear resistance of silicone impression materials

E Addition-cured silicone materials shrink more than condensation-cured silicone impression materials

8.17 Cavity linings/bases are used to:

A Protect the pulp from chemical changes

B Protect the pulp from thermal changes

C Provide adhesion between the tooth and restoration

D Treat the pulp

E Provide insulation under a metallic restoration to maximise galvanic effects

8.18 Flow of luting material is increased by:

A Venting the restoration

B Applying greater force when seating the restoration

C Increasing the taper of the preparation

D Decreasing the powder content of the cement

E None of the above

8.16   ABC

Polyether impression materials have good dimensional stability under conditions of low humidity, but they are hydrophilic and will absorb water in humid conditions. Polysulphide impression materials have better tear resistance than silicone impression materials. As there is little or no by-product in the cross-linking reaction of addition-cured silicones they create a dimensionally stable impression compared with condensation cured materials.

8.17   ABD

Cavity linings/bases act as a protective barrier between the dentine and the restoration. They may provide thermal insulation and chemical protection. They do provide insulation under metallic restorations – to minimise galvanic action. They do not provide adhesion between the tooth and the restoration.

8.18   ACD

Decreasing the powder content of a cement will make it less viscous and so it will increase the flow of the material. Application of greater force while seating will not increase the flow of luting material. Increasing the taper allows easier escape of luting material and hence increased flow.

8.19   With respect to acid etching:

A   It creates a microscopically rough enamel surface

B   Following etching the etchant should be washed away with saline

C   Enamel of deciduous teeth should be etched for a shorter time than permanent teeth

D   The etchant is usually 20% phosphoric acid

E   The etchant is usually applied for 15–30 seconds

8.20   Dentine bonding agents function by:

A   Micromechanical bonds

B   Macromechanical bonds

C   Primary atomic bonds

D   Secondary atomic bonds

E   All of the above

8.21   With regard to dental composite filling materials:

A   They consist of three phases: resin, organic filler particles and a coupling agent coated on the filler particles

B   The resin may be based on bis-GMA (dimethacrylate) oligomers

C   Macrofilled composites contain particles of about 0.5–2 μm in diameter

D   They usually contain fluoride

E   Microfilled composites are harder to polish than macrofilled composites

8.19 AE

The etchant is usually 30–50% phosphoric acid, which is applied for 15–30 seconds and creates a microscopically rough surface. As the enamel on deciduous teeth is not as regularly arranged as that on permanent teeth, they may need a longer etching time. The etchant is washed away with water not saline.

8.20 AD

Micromechanical bonds refer to the resin tags locking into the dentinal tubules. Secondary atomic bonding occurs as collagen and primers have polar groups attached to the main chains.

8.21 B

Composites consist of three phases: resin, inorganic filler particles and a coupling agent coated on the filler particles. Macrofilled composites have filler particles of around 2.5 –5 μm whereas microfilled composites have filler particles of about 0.04 μm in size. Glass ionomers, not composites, contain fluoride. The size of the filler particles determines the surface smoothness and hence microfilled composites tend to retain their shine longer and are easier to polish.

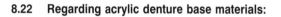

8.22 Regarding acrylic denture base materials:

A   They come in the form of a powder of polymethylmethacrylate and a liquid of ethylmethacrylate

B   An inhibitor such as benzyl peroxide is used to increase the shelf-life of the liquid

C   The material shrinks on setting

D   Heat curing leads to greater porosity in the material than cold curing

E   Ideally a high degree of conversion from monomer to polymer is desirable to increase mechanical properties of the material

8.23 Regarding the properties of casting gold alloys:

A   The gold content decreases on going from a soft type I alloy to an extra hard type IV alloy

B   The corrosion resistance increases on going from a soft type I alloy to an extra hard type IV alloy

C   The strength increases on going from a soft type I alloy to an extra hard type IV alloy

D   The ductility increases on going from a soft type I alloy to an extra hard type IV alloy

E   None of the above statements is correct

8.24 Regarding metals:

A   A molten metal should be cooled slowly to get a fine grain structure

B   Cold working will increase hardness and strength of a metal

C   Cold working will increase the brittleness of a metal

D   Internal stresses of a cold-worked metal may be removed by heat treatment at a temperature above the crystallisation temperature

E   Internal stresses of a cold-worked metal may be removed by heat treatment at a temperature below the crystallisation temperature

8.22 CE

Acrylic denture materials are usually formed of polymethylmethacrylate, which is formed by polymerisation of methylmethacrylate. They come in the form of a powder of polymethylmethacrylate and a liquid of methylmethacrylate. An inhibitor such as hydroquinone is used to increase the shelf-life of the liquid. Benzyl peroxide is the initiator, not the inhibitor. The material shrinks by about 20% on setting. Heat curing leads to less porosity in the material than cold curing. Low molecular polymer and residual monomer in the material lead to poor mechanical properties and sometime adverse tissue reactions.

8.23 AC

Type I soft casting gold alloys have about 85% gold whereas extra-hard type IV alloys have about 65% gold. This alters the properties of the alloy and the corrosion resistance and the ductility decrease on going from a soft type I alloy to an extra-hard type IV alloy.

8.24 BCE

A molten metal should be cooled rapidly to get a fine grain structure. Internal stresses of a cold-worked metal may be removed by heat treatment at a temperature well below the crystallisation temperature.

8.25 **Regarding casting faults:**

A   Incomplete casting could occur if the alloy is not properly melted

B   Incomplete casting may occur if there is insufficient thrust during casting

C   In order to limit porosity of a cast all casting moulds should be handled with the sprue downwards

D   Finning occurs when the investment is heated up too slowly

E   Porosity may be reduced by avoiding overheating of the alloy

8.25 ABCE

To limit porosity of a cast all casting moulds should be handled with the sprue downwards, otherwise broken bits of investment or dirt may fall down the sprue and become embedded in the casting. Handling moulds with the sprue directed downwards will limit this. Finning occurs when the investment is heated up too fast and cracks occur in the investment. Molten alloy flows into the cracks and creates fins on the casting.

9

Radiology and Radiography

9.1   Which of the following statements are correct?

A   A patient presents to your practice with chronic pain in the lower left third molar tooth. Examination reveals a mesio-angularly partially erupted, carious lower left third molar. The only other finding of note is caries in the upper left third molar. A full mouth dental panoramic radiograph would be your radiograph of choice

B   A patient presents with a retained upper left deciduous canine. An upper standard occlusal radiograph would be the radiograph of choice as it will give all the information that is needed about the deciduous tooth and the bucco-palatal position of an unerupted permanent canine if it is present

C   A patient has meal time syndrome and a palpable mass in the floor of the mouth. A lower standard occlusal radiograph may give you more information as to the cause of the meal time syndrome

D   A patient presents with dull aching pain across the mid part of their face which is worse on bending forward. An occipito-mental radiograph should be taken if you suspect sinusitis

E   In order to accurately visualise the interior dental nerve to allow the surgical removal of a lower third molar tooth a periapical radiograph and a dental panoramic radiograph must be taken.

9.2   A 30-year-old patient presents with a radiolucency at the angle of the mandible. Which of the following statements are correct?

A   In a white patient the lesion would not be an ameloblastoma

B   If the lesion is unilocular it is not a keratocyst (keratocystic odontogenic tumour)

C   If the lesion is well defined and unilocular and lies below the inferior dental canal it is likely to be Stafne's bone cavity

D   If the lesion is well defined and unilocular and lies below the inferior dental canal it is likely to be a solitary bone cyst

E   The lesion is likely to be a giant cell lesion as the angle of the mandible is the commonest location for this lesion

9.1   C

In the first patient, as there is disease only on the left hand side of the mouth there is no indication to irradiate both sides of the mouth. Hence a sectional panoramic radiograph would be adequate or even two periapical views. In the second patient, a standard occlusal view would be indicated, but on its own it will not give you accurate information on the bucco-palatal position of the underlying permanent canine tooth if one is present. Taking another radiograph would enable you to carry out the parallax technique and accurately locate an impacted tooth.

Although an occipito-mental radiograph will give you information on the maxillary antra, it is not considered necessary nowadays to take an occipito-mental radiograph to reach a diagnosis of sinusitis, as this is a clinical diagnosis. In the last scenario, one radiographic view that has good definition and shows the root and inferior dental canal is considered adequate prior to the surgical removal of a lower third molar.

9.2   C

Ameloblastomas are the commonest odontogenic tumours and can occur in any ethnic group although are more common in black Afro-Caribbean males. Odontogenic keratocysts (keratocystic odontogenic tumours) are often multilocular but unilocular ones do occur. Stafne's bone cavity is thought to be a depression on the lingual aspect of the mandible that contains aberrant salivary gland tissue, hence it is seen below the inferior dental canal.

Solitary bone cysts often occur in young adults, usually less than 25 and appear as radiolucent areas that extend up between the roots of the teeth. Giant cell lesions do occur in young adults but they are rare and are usually seen in the anterior mandible, often crossing the midline.

9.3 **You have taken a periapical radiograph and the resulting film is very pale. Which of the following may have caused this problem?**

A The film is overexposed

B The film is underexposed

C The developer was too hot

D The developer was contaminated by fixer

E The developer was too dilute

9.4 **Which of the following would cause the film fault described below?**

A A patient who moved during the exposure may cause the image to appear blurred on the film

B A patient who is excessively thin may cause a film to appear too dark

C If a film that was out of date was used it may cause the image to appear foggy

D If there was a fault in the processing unit or dark room that allowed ingress of light the film would appear too pale

E An image may appear blurred if a film was bent excessively during the exposure

9.3 BDE

Pale films may be caused by underexposure or by underdevelopment, which can occur if the developer is too cold, too weak or contaminated by the fixer.

9.4 ABCE

Stray light in a dark room or processing unit will make a film appear foggy.

9.5 **Which of the following are principles of the International Commission for Radiation Protection (ICRP)?**

  A Personal monitoring

  B Limitation

  C Screening

  D Justification

  E Optimisation

9.6 **Which of the following procedures may be undertaken by a registered dental nurse who has been appropriately trained?**

  A Reception and clerical duties

  B Taking of long cone periapical radiographs

  C Placement of temporary restorations in adults

  D Placement of temporary restorations in children

  E Impression taking

9.7 **You have taken a radiograph to assess a lower third molar for surgical removal. Which of the following radiological features would suggest that the patient would be at high risk of suffering from damage to their inferior dental nerve during the removal of the lower third molar tooth?**

  A Loss of tramlines of the inferior dental canal

  B Deviation of tramlines of the inferior dental canal

  C Widening of tramlines of the inferior dental canal

  D Narrowing of tramlines of the inferior dental canal

  E Radiopaque band across root

9.5   BDE

The ICRP recommendations are based on the principles of justification, optimisation and limitation.

- Justification – no practice should be adopted unless it produces a net benefit.
- Optimisation – all exposures should be kept as low as reasonably possible (ALARP).
- Limitation – the dose equivalent should not exceed the recommended limits.

9.6   AB

To take radiographs dental nurses should possess a certificate in dental radiography from a course conforming to the syllabus prescribed by the College of Radiographers.

9.7   ABD

Loss, narrowing and deviation of the tramlines of the inferior dental canal are all taken as evidence of association of the inferior dental nerve with a lower molar tooth. A radiolucent band across the root is also thought to indicate association of the nerve and tooth. Hence patients with these radiological features are at high risk of inferior dental nerve damage during surgical removal of lower third molar teeth.

9.8 **Everyday risks to patients having radiographs taken during the course of their dental treatment include:**

    A   Genetic stochastic effects

    B   Somatic stochastic effects

    C   Somatic deterministic effects

    D   Genetic deterministic effects

    E   None of the above

9.9 **In order to limit the dose for a periapical radiograph:**

    A   Use a lead apron

    B   Use a bisecting angle technique

    C   Use a low-speed film

    D   Use the optimal voltage (70 kV)

    E   Use a rectangular collimator

9.10 **With respect to processing radiographs:**

    A   The developer is an acidic solution

    B   The developer is oxidised by air and so must be changed daily

    C   If the film is left in the developer for too long it will result in a radiograph being too pale/light

    D   The lower the temperature of the developer solution the faster the film will be developed

    E   Fixation involves the unsensitised silver halide crystals being removed to reveal the white areas on the film

9.8 ABC

Stochastic effects are random, and can be divided into somatic and genetic. Deterministic effects are only somatic.

9.9 DE

Use of lead aprons is no longer recommended. To minimise the risk the optimal voltage (70 kV) and a fast-speed film should be used. A rectangular collimator will reduce the radiation by about 50% compared with a round collimator.

9.10 E

The developer is an alkali solution, which is oxidised by air, but is usually changed about once every 10–14 days. If the film is left in it for too long it will become too dark as more silver will be deposited on it. The higher the temperature of the developer solution the faster the process will occur – the norm is 5 minutes at 20 °C.

9.11 **The stages of processing of radiographic films are:**

A Development, washing, fixation, washing, drying

B Fixation, washing, development, washing drying

C Washing, development, washing, fixation, drying

D Washing, fixation, washing, development, drying

E Washing development, fixation, washing drying

9.12 **All dental practices should have a set of local rules relating to radiation protection measures. These should include:**

A The name of the radiation protection supervisor (RPS)

B Contact details of the RPS

C Identification and description of the controlled area

D Arrangements for pregnant staff

E Qualifications of the RPS

9.13 **The annual dose limits under the Ionising Radiation Regulations (IRR) 1999 are:**

A General public – 2 mSv

B Non-classified workers – 5 mSv

C Non-classified workers – 6 mSv

D Classified workers – 20 mSv

E Classified workers – 60 mSv

9.11 A

When placed in the developer the sensitised silver halide crystals on the film are chemically reduced to black metallic silver. The film is then washed to remove the excess developer and placed in the fixer where the unsensitised silver halide crystals are removed, revealing the transparent parts of the image. The film is washed to remove excess fixer solution and dried.

9.12 ACD

All dental practices should have a set of local rules regarding radiation protection measures. The contact details of the RPS are not needed as they work at the practice, nor are their qualifications necessary.

9.13 CD

The annual dose limits according to IRR 1999 are:

- Classified workers – 20m Sv
- Non-classified workers – 6 mSv
- General public 1 – mSv

9.14 **Film badges for monitoring and measuring radiation dosage:**

  A Provide a permanent record of dose received

  B Should be worn outside the clothes at the level of the reproductive organs

  C Can measure the type and energy of radiation encountered

  D Can be assessed without processing so provide an immediate indication of exposure

  E Should be replaced every 6 months

9.15 **Regarding thermoluminescent dosimeters:**

  A They are used for monitoring radiation dose of the whole body

  B They can provide a permanent record of dose received

  C They use a material which absorbs radiation and then releases the energy in the form of light

  D The monitor should be replaced after 1–3 months

  E An advantage they have over film badges is that the monitor does not need to be replaced so frequently

9.16 **The advantages of the paralleling technique of periapical radiography over the bisecting angle technique are:**

  A It is possible to get reproducible radiographs, even when different operators take them

  B No film holder is needed

  C The image produced shows little or no magnification

  D The film is not coned off

  E Positioning the film to take radiographs of posterior teeth is usually comfortable for the patient

9.14   ABC

Film badges are a simple and inexpensive way of recording radiation exposure. The film is usually worn outside the clothes at the level of the reproductive organs for 1–3 months. It is then processed to reveal a permanent record of the radiation dose received; no information can be gained until the film is processed, and so these badges are prone to processing errors.

9.15   ACD

Thermoluminescent dosimeters are personal monitors that contain a material that absorbs radiation and releases energy in the form of light proportional to the amount of radiation received. They are worn like a film badge and should be replaced every 1–3 months. They do not provide a permanent record, and so cannot be stored and rechecked.

9.16   ACD

As film holders are used to take periapical radiographs in the paralleling technique it is possible to get reproducible radiographs. However, positioning the film for posterior teeth may sometimes be uncomfortable.

9.17 **Which of the following are indications to take a lower occlusal radiograph?**

A   To detect a salivary calculus in the parotid duct

B   To assess fractures in the anterior body of the mandible

C   To assess the buccolingual position of unerupted maxillary teeth

D   To assess any buccolingual expansion of the anterior mandible by pathological lesions

E   To assess the buccolingual position of unerupted mandibular third molars

9.18 **Which of the following could present as multilocular radiolucent lesions in the mandible?**

A   Ameloblastoma

B   Calcifying epithelial odontogenic tumour

C   Odontogenic keratocyst (keratocystic odontogenic tumours)

D   Odontogenic myxoma

E   Aneurysmal bone cyst

9.19 **Which of the following lesions could present as a unilocular radiolucent lesion in the mandible?**

A   Dentigerous cyst

B   Ameloblastoma

C   Ameloblastic fibroma

D   Residual cyst

E   Stafne's bone cavity

9.17   BD

A lower occlusal radiograph can show a calculus in the submandibular gland duct but not in the parotid. It will show any buccolingual displacement of a symphyseal or parasymphyseal fracture of the mandible and buccolingual expansion of the mandible in the anterior mandible. It is not used to assess the buccolingual position of unerupted third molars.

9.18   ACDE

Calcifying epithelial odontogenic tumours are not usually radiolucent but are radiopaque due to the calcifying nature of the lesion.

9.19   ABCDE

Dentigerous cysts, residual cysts and Stafne's bone cavities all appear as unilocular radiolucent lesions on radiographs. Stafre's bone cavities are only seen below the inferior dental canal. Ameloblastomas although often multilocular may appear as unilocular lesions. Keratocysts (keratocystic odontogenic tumours) are also usually multilocular, but may appear unilocular in the early stages.

9.20 Which of the following lesions could present as a radiopaque lesion in the mandible on a dental panoramic tomogram (DPT)?

A Calcifying epithelial odontogenic tumour

B Complex odontoma

C Odontogenic fibroma

D Cemento-osseous dysplasia

E Submandibular gland calculus

9.21 An ideal radiograph produces an image in which the size and shape of the object (tooth) is reproduced exactly on the film, without distortion or magnification. To produce an image as close to this which of the following principles must be applied?

A The distance between the tube and the film should be as small as possible

B The distance between the film and the object should be as small as possible

C The film should lie as near to parallel to the tooth as is possible

D The beam should be as near to perpendicular to the tooth as possible

E The patient should hold their breath during the taking of the radiograph

9.20 ABDE

All of the above lesions except an odontogenic fibroma could appear as radiopaque lesions in the mandible.

9.21 BCD

The distance between the tube and the film should be as large as possible. It is not necessary for patients to hold their breath during the taking of the radiograph but the patient, the tube and the film should be motionless.

10

Restorative
Dentistry

10.1 **Which of the following statements regarding the dental chart shown below are correct?**

A   The patient has a disto-occlusal amalgam filling in the upper left second premolar

B   The patient has a disto-occlusal amalgam filling in the upper right second premolar

C   The patient has a mesio-occlusal amalgam filling in the upper left second premolar

D   The patient has a mesio-occlusal amalgam filling in the upper right second premolar

E   The patient has a buccal cervical cavity in the upper left canine

10.2 **Which of the following statements regarding the dental chart below are correct?**

A   The patient has had the lower left third molar extracted

B   The patient needs to have the lower left third molar extracted

C   The patient has an occluso-buccal amalgam restoration in the lower right first permanent molar

D   The patient has an occluso-buccal cavity in the lower right first permanent molar

E   The patient has an occluso-buccal temporary restoration in the lower right first permanent molar

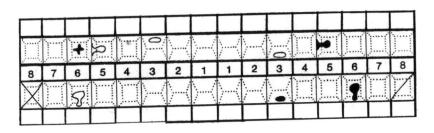

10.1   C

The patient has a mesio-occlusal amalgam filling in the upper left second premolar, and a disto-occlusal cavity in the upper right second premolar. There is a palatal cervical cavity in the upper left canine and a labial cervical cavity in the upper right canine.

10.2   BD

The patient has had the lower right third molar tooth extracted. The patient has an occluso-buccal amalgam restoration in the lower left first permanent molar.

10.3 **When planning dental treatment, principles of aesthetic dentistry are important. Which of the following statements regarding aesthetic dentistry are correct?**

A The so called 'golden proportion' is a ratio between height and width. The golden proportion of 1.5:1 of height to width ratio of incisors is aimed for, as this is thought to be aesthetically pleasing

B When considering the symmetry of a patient's dentition the width of the teeth is more noticeable than the height, which is more noticeable than the depth of the teeth

C When considering the symmetry of a patient's dentition the depth is more important than the height, which is more noticeable than width of teeth

D Black triangles, which appear with loss of gingival tissue, are much more noticeable in patients with low smile lines than high smile lines

E The desirable maxillary gingival contour has the highest gingival margin over the central incisor, followed by the canine and then the lateral incisor

10.4 **Appropriate basic periodontal treatment in general dental practice should include:**

A Patient motivation

B Anti-smoking advice

C Periodontal surgery

D Three-monthly bitewing radiographs to show bone levels

E Removal of plaque retentive factors

10.3   B

The 'golden proportion' is often aimed for with regards to height to width ratio of teeth but it is 1.6:1 not 1.5:1. Harmony in a smile/dentition is related to symmetry and width of teeth is more important than height of teeth, which is more important than depth of teeth. Black triangles are formed when the interdental papillae are lost and they form an aesthetic problem when they are most visible. Patients with high smile lines are more likely to show black triangles on anterior maxillary teeth than those with low smile lines. Hence, it is more of an aesthetic problem in patients with high smile lines. The ideal gingival contour of the anterior maxillary region is often described as having a 'gull wing' appearance. For an ideal appearance the gingival contour of the canine should be slightly higher than the gingival margin of the central incisor, which should be slightly higher than the contour of the lateral incisor. For the best appearance the two sides should be symmetrical.

10.4   ABE

A minimum standard of basic periodontal treatment should be given to all patients who require it in general practice. It should include patient motivation, oral hygiene instruction and advice about smoking cessation. Removal of supragingival and subgingival deposits should also be undertaken along with removal of plaque retentive factors. All treatment should be monitored to see what progress has been made. Periodontal surgery is more complex and may need referral to a specialist. Bitewing radiographs should not be taken at three-monthly intervals. Radiographs are indicated when there is clinical evidence that the disease is progressing.

10.5 **In which of the following scenarios would a shortened dental arch be contraindicated?**

A A patient aged 52 with evidence of parafunction or abnormal wear

B A patient aged 55 with a centric stop on the canines with stable posterior contacts as far back as the second premolars

C A 45-year-old patient with an anterior open bite

D A 49-year-old patient with a class 1 malocclusion and pre-existing temporomandibular disorder

E A 56-year-old patient with a class 1 malocclusion and progressive caries confined to the molars

10.6 **A patient needs an increase in vertical dimension as part of their restorative treatment plan. Which of the following would be a sensible way to proceed?**

A Provide the patient with an appliance with an anterior bite plane to wear while eating to see if they can tolerate the increased vertical dimension

B Provide the patient with an appliance with an anterior bite plane to wear in the evening and overnight

C Provide the patient with a Michigan splint to wear while eating

D Provide the patient with a Michigan splint to wear in the evening and overnight

E Increase the vertical dimension, and if the patient develops symptoms provide them with a bite raising appliance

10.7 **Hypodontia**
Which of the following may predispose a patient to hypodontia?

A Cleidocranial dysplasia

B Down's syndrome

C Ectodermal dysplasia

D Gorlin–Goltz syndrome/multiple basal cell naevi syndrome

E Gardener's syndrome

10.5 ACD

A shortened dental arch is considered acceptable especially in older patients and when the patient has stable posterior contacts as far back as the second premolars or first molars and the anterior teeth have a favourable prognosis. It is not indicated in patients under the age of 50 with anterior open bites or pre-existing abnormal parafunctional habits, excessive tooth wear or temporomandibular problems.

10.6 B

To ensure a patient can tolerate an increase in the occlusal vertical dimension it is common to give them an appliance to wear for several weeks and over 12 hours at each time; if there are no masticatory muscle or temporomandibular joint problems it is usually safe to proceed. The appliance may have an anterior bite plane, or be full coverage. Care needs to be taken if the splint used is partial coverage as long-term wear may cause over-eruption of other teeth.

A Michigan splint is a full coverage maxillary stabilisation splint that provides stable intercuspal position contacts between a generally flat surface and the opposing teeth, which causes the anterior teeth to be out of contact. It is used to treat temporomandibular problems.

10.7 BC

In cleidocranial dysplasia, the patient often has multiple supernumerary teeth. Gorlin–Goltz syndrome (multiple basal cell naevi syndrome) consists of multiple keratocysts (odontogenic keratocystic tumours), multiple basal cell carcinomas, bifid ribs, frontal bossing, calcified falx cerebri and skeletal abnormalities. Gardener's syndrome consists of multiple osteomas, intestinal polyps and epidermoid cysts.

10.8 **Which of the following are not indications for crown lengthening procedures?**

A   To relocate the margins of restorations that are impinging on biological width

B   To access supragingival caries

C   To produce a ferrule for post crown provision

D   To increase the clinical crown height that has been lost due to caries or tooth wear

E   To gain access to a perforation in the apical third of the root

10.9 **Which of the following should be taken into consideration when planning cavity preparation for a posterior composite?**

A   Bevelling is recommended on the occlusal surface to enable a thin margin of composite to flow onto sound tooth structure

B   Internal line angles should be rounded where ever possible to reduce stress concentration in the material

C   Interproximal boxes should be extended so that the cervical margin is below the contact point and the vertical margins are buccal and lingual to the contact points

D   The cavity preparation should follow the fissure pattern but should not be extended into sound fissures

E   Enamel should be preserved at the cavity margins and on the cervical floor of the box as this will allow better seal of the material than would be achieved if the margins were in dentine

10.10 **You are examining a patient whom you suspect has a cracked tooth. Which of the following signs and symptoms and diagnostic tests would help confirm your diagnosis?**

A   The patient has pain when they bite on something

B   The patient has pain when they release their bite

C   The tooth is tender to percussion

D   Applying an orthodontic band to the tooth results in a reduction in the pain

E   Transillumination shows that light travels through the tooth

10.8   BE

Crown lengthening is indicated in many situations and depends on a variety of dental and patient related factors. It can be carried out to increase clinical crown height, gain access to subgingival caries and to reposition margins of restorations above the gingival margin. Any restoration that impinges on the biological width (which is the distance from the crest of the alveolar bone to the gingival margin) is thought to have an adverse effect on periodontal health. It can also be used to gain access to root perforations but usually in the coronal third of the root.

10.9   BDE

Occlusal forces may fracture a thin layer of occlusal composite which would be present if the margins were bevelled, hence bevelling is not recommended on the occlusal surface. The vertical margins of the interproximal box do not have to be buccal and lingual to the contact point, they may be left in contact so long as it is possible to adapt the matrix band. Composites have a better bond strength to enamel than dentine and degrade less with time so keeping margins on enamel will create a restoration that is less likely to fail.

10.10   BD

Cracked teeth tend to cause pain when pressure on them is relieved, and more specifically when pressure on individual cusps is relieved. They are not always tender to percussion as it depends where the pressure is applied – if the pressure does not cause separation of the cracked pieces it may not evoke pain. Holding the cracked pieces together with orthodontic bands may reduce the pain. Transillumination will allow light to travel through the tooth up to the crack.

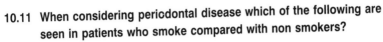

10.11 When considering periodontal disease which of the following are seen in patients who smoke compared with non smokers?

   A Smokers tend to have increased gingival inflammation and bleeding

   B Smoking is thought to have an effect on local erythrocyte function and this is a possible reason for the increased risk/prevalence of periodontal disease in smokers

   C Poorer plaque control in smokers is thought to contribute to their increased risk/prevalence of periodontal disease

   D Studies has conclusively shown that smoking always affects the microbial composition of the plaque, leading to an increased risk/prevalence of periodontal disease

   E The number of cigarettes smoked per day has no bearing on the severity of the disease, it is only the length of time that the patient has smoked for that has an effect

10.12 Enamel microabrasion would be useful to treat which the following conditions that may cause teeth to be discoloured?

   A Enamel decalcification defects left after removal of fixed orthodontic brackets

   B Dentinogenesis imperfecta

   C Tetracycline staining

   D Amelogenesis imperfecta

   E White discoloration caused by fluorosis

10.11   All statements are false

Smokers tend to have less gingival inflammation and bleeding than non-smokers. The increased susceptibility to periodontal disease in smokers is not thought to be due to poorer plaque control, and there is some controversy over the effect of smoking on the microbial composition of plaque. Smoking has been shown to affect neutrophil function, not erythrocyte function. Both the number of cigarettes smoked per day and the length of time smoked will have a bearing on the periodontal status.

10.12   AE

Enamel microabrasion is a technique that involves both abrasion and erosion and removes the surface enamel. It is good for removing stains/discolouration from the surface of enamel, but not intrinsic staining. The discolouration in dentinogenesis imperfecta and in tetracycline staining is within the dentine and in amelogenesis imperfect the discolouration is within the enamel rather than on the surface of the enamel.

10.13 **Which of the following statements regarding electrosurgery used for restorative dentistry in the dental surgery are correct?**

A Electrosurgery can be used for gingival retraction prior to taking impressions, and is very useful in situations where the tissues have a thin biotype

B The results achieved are equally good in cases where gingival inflammation is present as in those without gingival inflammation

C Electrosurgery can be used to increase crown height and hence the surface area available for bonding of a resin bonded bridge retainer

D As electrosurgery units use only low-frequency electrical energy it is possible to use metallic instruments while carrying out electrosurgery

E Post-operative pain experienced by patients following electrosurgical procedures is usually mild but analgesics may be required

10.14 **The following are indications for flowable resin composites:**

A As a cavity liner

B Restoring deciduous teeth

C Preventive resin restorations

D As a retrograde root filling material

E To block out undercuts in inlay preparations

10.15 **Conventional resin-retained bridges have a metal framework, but newer techniques with fibre-reinforced composite have been developed. The following are advantages of a fibre-reinforced resin-retained bridge:**

A Better aesthetics as the framework is tooth coloured

B Less space for occlusal clearance is needed

C They can be fabricated by a direct or indirect method

D The bond of the composite retainers to the etched enamel is thought to be more reliable than that to the metal retainers

E The fibre components can be arranged to provide strength in areas where it is needed

10.13 CE

Electrosurgery can be used for gingival retraction prior to taking impressions, but care must be taken in situations where the tissues have a thin biotype. It can be used in cases where gingival inflammation is present but better results are often achieved if the gingival tissues are healthy and inflammation-free prior to the surgery. Electrosurgery units use high-frequency electrical energy hence use of metallic instruments may result in a conductive burn. To avoid this, the use of plastic instruments is recommended.

10.14 ABCE

Commonly used retrograde filling materials are MTA (mineral trioxide aggregate), IRM® and glass ionomer cement.

10.15 ACDE

Fibre-reinforced resin-retained bridges are relatively new and so long-term data on their performance is not yet available. However, it is thought that although the bond strengths and strength of the materials will be adequate, more space is needed for occlusal clearance of the retainer. This is because the material is not as strong as conventional metallic frameworks.

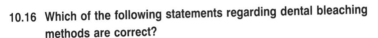

10.16 Which of the following statements regarding dental bleaching methods are correct?

A   All bleaching agents work via the action of hydrogen dioxide

B   Bleaching agents break down rapidly into free radicals and oxygen, which act to break down the large molecules causing discolouration into smaller molecules

C   Possible complications of bleaching include sensitivity of teeth and gingival irritation

D   The concentration of bleaching agent used is 30% for all types of vital bleaching

E   Some degree of shade regression is normal with all types of bleaching

10.17 Root caries:

A   Is commoner in patients with reduced salivary flow than those with a normal salivary flow

B   Is commoner in females than in males

C   Is often managed with topical fluoride

D   Is often managed with systemic fluoride

E   May be managed by surface recontouring without a restoration

10.18 The following statements are correct:

A   The Bennett angle is the mean angle between the sagittal plane and the path of the advancing condyle during lateral excursions as viewed in the horizontal plane

B   The condylar angle is the angle between the horizontal plane and the distal slope of the articular eminence

C   The curve of Spee is the curvature of the occlusion viewed in the coronal plane

D   The curve of Wilson is the curvature of the occlusion viewed in the sagittal plane

E   Retruded contact position is the initial tooth contact when the mandible rotates around its terminal hinge axis

10.16 BCE

The active agent in all bleaching systems is hydrogen peroxide, as carbamide peroxide and sodium perborate are all broken down to hydrogen peroxide. Sensitivity of teeth and gingival irritation has been reported with bleaching but both are thought to be reversible. Gingival irritation is thought to occur most commonly when high concentrations of bleaching agent are used.

Different concentrations of bleaching agent are used, depending on the method of vital bleaching. For example, bleaching in the dental surgery requires high concentrations (up to 35%) of hydrogen peroxide, whereas home bleaching kits usually contain 10% carbamide peroxide gel.

Shade regression is normal following the end of bleaching and patients should be warned of this. In addition, any final restorations should delayed for a couple of weeks post bleaching.

10.17 ACE

Root caries is a common complication of dry mouth. The lesions are often managed with topical fluoride. Systemic fluoride is not suitable as the teeth are already formed. The lesions may be managed by recontouring without placement of a restoration if they are small. Larger ones are often filled with glass ionomer cement.

10.18 ABE

The curve of Spee is the curvature of the occlusion viewed in the sagittal plane and the curve of Wilson is the curvature of the occlusion viewed in the coronal plane.

10.19 You are planning on restoring an upper first premolar with a porcelain restoration. Which of the following would be indications to extend the porcelain coverage over the occlusal surface of the tooth?

A Aesthetics

B The tooth is very short in height

C The tooth has a large pulp cavity

D The opposing teeth have porcelain occlusal coverage

E The tooth is heavily restored

10.20 With respect to crown preparations:

A Resistance refers to resistance to dislodgement of the restoration under oblique forces

B Resistance refers to resistance to dislodgement of the restoration under forces in the path of insertion of the restoration

C Retention refers to resistance to dislodgement of the restoration under oblique forces

D Retention refers to resistance to dislodgement of the restoration under forces in the path of insertion of the restoration

E Height and taper of the preparation are major features in both resistance and retention

10.21 You are restoring a vital lower first permanent molar with a deep carious cavity. In order to minimise the risk of bacteria gaining access to the pulp you could plan to:

A Carry out indirect pulp capping

B Carry out direct pulp capping

C Remove caries from the cavity wall before the cavity floor

D Remove caries from the floor of the cavity before the cavity walls

E Give the patient a course of antibiotics for a week

10.19 ADE

Metal occlusal coverage requires less tooth tissue removal and is therefore indicated when teeth are short and have large pulps. Porcelain occlusal coverage can be used when aesthetics is critical, when teeth are heavily restored and when they will occlude against porcelain.

10.20 ADE

Resistance refers to features that prevent removal or dislodgement of the restoration under oblique forces. Retention refers to features that that prevent removal or dislodgement of the restoration under forces along the long axis.

10.21 AC

The rationale behind indirect pulp capping is that demineralisation of the dentine precedes bacterial invasion. Hence it is possible to remove the infected dentine and treat the demineralised dentine with a base layer to encourage remineralisation.

You would not plan to do direct pulp capping as this would expose the pulp and increase the likelihood of bacteria gaining access to it. Caries should always be removed from the cavity walls first so that if an exposure is made there is a minimal load of infected material in the cavity to infect the pulp.

10.22 A water spray is used with rotary instruments to:

 A   Reduce heating of the dentine

 B   Reduce clogging of burs

 C   Minimise movement of fluid in dentinal tubules

 D   Remove debris away from operative site

 E   Allow potentially infectious body fluid to be aspirated rather than creating an aerosol

10.23 Which of the following statements about tooth surface wear are correct?

 A   Attrition is tooth surface wear by non-bacterial chemical dissolution

 B   Abrasion is tooth surface wear by other teeth

 C   Abrasion is tooth surface wear by surfaces other than teeth

 D   Erosion is tooth surface wear by non-bacterial chemical dissolution

 E   Erosion is tooth surface wear by surfaces other than teeth

10.24 Regarding non-carious tooth surface loss:

 A   Abrasion is characterised by smooth wear facets

 B   Abrasion is the commonest type of tooth wear in young patients

 C   'Cupped out' concavities are seen in patients with erosion

 D   Abfraction is due to stresses around the cervical margins due to flexure of teeth

 E   Erosion by gastric acid is usually seen on the labial aspect of the upper teeth

10.25 Which of the following are methods of monitoring tooth surface loss?

 A   Dietary sheets

 B   Study models

 C   Smith and Kidd indices

 D   Laser scanning

 E   Clinical photographs

10.22 ABD

The water spray minimises damage to pulpal tissue via desiccation of dentine. It also helps to prevent the burs from becoming clogged. It does not minimise fluid movement in dentinal tubules. It has the detrimental effect of causing an aerosol which is potentially infectious.

10.23 CD

Tooth surface wear by non-bacterial chemical dissolution (dietary or gastric acid) is erosion, tooth surface wear by other teeth is attrition and tooth surface wear by surfaces other than teeth is abrasion.

10.24 CD

Attrition is the loss of tooth substance due to tooth–tooth contact and causes smooth wear facets. Abrasion is the wear of substance from an external agent, eg buccal cervical notches caused by toothbrushing, although other factors may also be operating. It is often seen in older patients. Erosion is the commonest type of tooth wear seen in young patients and when caused by gastric acid it is usually seen on the palatal aspect of the maxillary teeth.

Abfraction is due to stresses around the cervical margin due to flexure of the root and crown of the tooth. This causes minute cracks to propagate under occlusal forces.

10.25 BDE

Smith and Knight tooth indices are used to monitor tooth wear. Dietary sheets are useful to determine the cause of the problem. Laser and computer scanning of the study models and dentition – as with the other methods – taken over a period of time can be used to monitor the progression of the condition.

10.26 **Which of the following may be signs and symptoms of reversible pulpitis?**

   A   Pain on biting

   B   Sensitivity on application of heat

   C   Sensitivity on application of sweet

   D   Well localised pain

   E   Poorly localised pain

10.27 **Which of the following may be signs and symptoms of irreversible pulpitis?**

   A   Pain on application of heat

   B   Well localised pain

   C   Poorly localised pain

   D   Spontaneous pain

   E   Sharp, shooting pain

10.28 **Which of the following statements about fluoride are true?**

   A   The safely tolerated dose of fluoride (ie the dose below which symptoms of toxicity are unlikely) is 1 mg/kg of body weight

   B   The safely tolerated dose of fluoride is 0.5 mg/kg of body weight

   C   The certainly lethal dose (ie the dose at which survival is unlikely) is 10–15 mg/kg body weight

   D   The certainly lethal dose is 15–20 mg/kg body weight

   E   The potentially lethal dose (ie the lowest dose associated with fatality) is 10 mg/kg body weight

10.26 BCE

Reversible pulpitis tends to cause poorly localised pain. Pain is elicited on application of hot, cold or sweet food but not on biting.

10.27 ABCD

In irreversible pulpitis there is usually spontaneous pain which may last from a few seconds to several hours. Heat causes pain which lasts long after the stimulus is withdrawn whereas cold sometimes actually relieves the pain. Irreversible pulpitis may be poorly localised if the periodontal ligament is not involved, but as soon as it is involved the patient will be able to localise the pain.

10.28 A

The potentially lethal dose of fluoride (ie the lowest dose associated with fatality) is 5 mg/kg body weight. The certainly lethal dose of fluoride (ie the dose at which survival is unlikely) is 32–64 mg/kg body weight. A person who has had a potentially lethal dose should be hospitalised.

10.29 The desirable degree of taper of a preparation to receive a cast restoration is:

    A   <2°

    B   2–4°

    C   5–7°

    D   8–12°

    E   >12°

10.30 Regarding porcelain veneers:

    A   They are more durable than composite veneers in terms of colour and surface gloss

    B   The occlusion is not usually affected as they do not cover the palatal aspect of the teeth

    C   They are less likely to fracture than composite veneers

    D   They are more conservative of tooth tissue than crown preparations

    E   They usually require no preparation of the labial surface

10.31 When considering pin placement for large restorations:

    A   The pins should be placed in the dentinoenamel junction

    B   The pins should be placed in dentine

    C   The more pins used the stronger the restoration will be

    D   When more than one pin is used they must be placed parallel to each other

    E   Pins should be placed about 2–2.5 mm into the remaining tooth structure

10.29   C

The more parallel the walls of a restoration the greater the resistance to displacement is. However, it is not possible to achieve exactly parallel walls and so a degree of taper is acceptable, the desired taper being about 5–7°.

10.30   ABD

Porcelain is brittle and likely to fracture. Porcelain veneers usually require some preparation of tooth tissue, but they are much more conservative than crown preparations.

10.31   BE

Pins should always be placed in dentine, not at the dentinoenamel junction as the undermined enamel may fracture away. The more pins that are placed the weaker the remaining tooth and restoration will be. Pins are usually placed at an angle to the cavity walls or to other pins if possible as this increases the resistance to dislodgement.

10.32 Which of the following statements are true?

A Enamel consists of 92% hydroxyapatite crystals by weight

B Enamel is thickest where it overlies the cusps of teeth

C Diamond burs remove enamel by fracturing it

D Tungsten carbide burs remove enamel by grinding

E Stresses within a cavity preparation can be minimised by rounding the internal line angles

10.33 Which of the following are desirable properties of a matrix band for use with amalgam restorations?

A The band provides a tight fit in the cervical region

B The width of the band should be such that it extends to the marginal ridge

C The band should be see-through to allow good visibility

D The band should be thin (approx 0.05 mm)

E The band should allow contact with the adjacent tooth to be re-established

10.34 Regarding the anatomy of root canals:

A A two-rooted lower first permanent molar usually has one canal in the mesial root and one canal in the distal root

B A two-rooted lower first permanent molar usually has two canals in the distal root and one in the mesial root

C A two-rooted lower first permanent molar usually has two canals in the mesial root and one in the distal root

D The palatal root is usually the longest root in a three-rooted maxillary first permanent molar

E The mesiobuccal root is usually longer than the palatal root in a three-rooted maxillary first permanent molar

10.32 BE

Enamel consists of 96–98% hydroxyapatite crystals by weight. It is thinnest buccally and thickest over the cusps of the teeth. Diamond burs remove enamel by grinding whereas tungsten carbide burs remove enamel by fracturing it.

10.33 ADE

Matrix bands need to provide a good fit in the cervical area and should extend to 1 mm above the marginal ridge to allow for over-packing of the cavity. Matrix bands for amalgam restorations are usually metallic and do not need to be see-through. They should be smooth, thin and be adaptable so the contact point with the adjacent tooth can be re-established.

10.34 CD

Two-rooted lower first permanent molars usually have two canals in the mesial root and one in the distal root. In three-rooted maxillary first permanent molars the palatal root is usually the longest root.

10.35 An ideal root canal filling material would have which of the following properties?

A   Non-irritant to the periapical tissues

B   Be radiolucent

C   Absorb moisture

D   Be easily introduced into the root canal system

E   Not visible through the dentine

10.36 Which of the following conditions may cause a root canal treatment to fail?

A   Bacteria left in accessory canals

B   Persistent infection of a root canal following treatment

C   Presence of a coronal restoration with inadequate margins

D   A vertical root fracture

E   Necrotic material being left in the canal during preparation

10.37 Obturation of a root canal system during root canal treatment aims to:

A   Provide a fluid-tight seal at the apical end of the root but not at the coronal end

B   Provide a fluid-tight seal at the coronal end of the root but not at the apical end

C   Provide a fluid-tight seal at both the apical and coronal ends of the root

D   Seal any remaining bacteria in the root canal system

E   Remove any remaining bacteria from the canal system

10.35   ADE

An ideal root canal filling material should be radio-opaque and should not absorb moisture – it should be impervious to moisture. The filler should not be visible through the coronal dentine.

10.36   ABCDE

All these conditions may cause failure of a root canal treatment.

10.37   CD

The aim of obturation is to provide a fluid-tight seal at both the apical and the coronal ends of the root canal. It also aims to seal any remaining bacteria in the canal system. Removal of bacteria is the aim of cleaning and preparing the canal.

10.38 Surgical endodontic treatment:

A   Is indicated for all failed root canal treatments

B   Is indicated when there is a broken instrument in the canal that cannot be bypassed

C   Is indicated to prevent removal of extensive coronal restorative work

D   Is indicated when there is evidence of a periapical radiolucency on radiographs

E   Is contra-indicated in all multi-rooted teeth

10.39 Which of the following are features of an access cavity?

A   It should only remove the roof of the pulp chamber over the entrance to the root canals

B   Provide unobstructed access to the root canals

C   Provide access in a straight line to the root canals

D   Have parallel or convergent walls to retain a temporary restoration

E   It is usually ovoid shaped for maxillary incisors

10.40 Which of the following are methods of obturating a canal with gutta percha?

A   Vertical condensation

B   Lateral trephination

C   Thermomechanical compaction

D   Using thermoplasticised gutta percha

E   Vertical trephination

10.38   BC

Orthograde root canal treatment is preferable to surgical endodontics as surgery only seals over the canal that has not been re-cleaned. However, surgical endodontics may be indicated when it is not possible to bypass a broken instrument or when conventional orthograde treatment would mean removal of extensive coronal restorative work. The presence of a periapical radiolucency on radiograph is not an indication for a surgical approach. Orthograde root canal treatments can cure periapical disease. It is possible to carry out surgical endodontics on multi-rooted teeth.

10.39   BC

An access cavity should not have any of the pulp chamber roof present, as this will get in the way of the access to the root canals. The walls should also be divergent, it is not necessary to have convergent walls to retain a restoration. It is usually triangular shaped for maxillary incisors.

10.40   ACD

Trephination means to cut a circular hole and has nothing to do with obturating root canals, hence vertical and lateral trephination do not exist.

10.41 Which of the following are true of pregnancy and gingival tissue:

A Oestrogen may stimulate growth of new blood vessels and increase vascular permeability leading to hyperaemic gingivitis

B Progesterone may stimulate growth of new blood vessels and increase vascular permeability leading to hyperaemic gingivitis

C Pregnancy is associated with modified inflammatory response resulting in fibrous gingival overgrowth

D High levels of progesterone increase the immune response to plaque

E High levels of oestrogen suppresse the immune response to plaque

10.42 Which of the following bacterial species are strongly associated with adult periodontitis?

A *Porphyromonas gingivalis*

B *Bacteroides forsythus*

C *Campylobacter rectus*

D *Treponema pallidum*

E *Prevotella intermedia*

10.43 The condition "aggressive periodontitis" (AgP) is characterised by:

A Rapid attachment loss

B Underlying medical condition

C Non-familial tendency

D Rapid bone destruction

E Patients below the age of 35 years

10.41   ABE

The elevated levels of progesterone and oestrogen in pregnancy are known to modulate vascular responses and connective tissue turnover in gingival tissues, resulting in pregnancy gingivitis. The high levels of progesterone and oestrogen in pregnancy also suppress the immune response to plaque. Drugs such as phenytoin, calcium-channel blockers, immunosuppressants, eg ciclosporin, are thought to modify the inflammatory response resulting in fibrous gingival overgrowth.

10.42   ABCE

Treponema pallidum is the organism responsible for syphilis. Besides the micro-organisms listed in the question, the following are also strongly associated with adult periodontitis: *Fusobacterium nucleatum*, *Actinomycetes actinomycetemcomitans*, *Eikenella corrodens*, *Eubacterium* species and spirochaetes, eg *Treponema denticola*.

10.43   AD

AgP comprises a group of severe rapidly progressive forms of periodontitis. It used to be called early-onset periodontitis (EOP), and can be divided into a localised form (previously localised juvenile periodontitis) and a generalised form (previously generalised juvenile periodontitis or generalised EOP). It is characterised by rapid attachment loss and bone destruction. There is no underlying medical condition and usually there is a familial tendency. It often affects young patients, but can occur at older ages as well, hence a cut off age of 35 years is not relevant.

10.44 **Which of the following functions of the predominant inflammatory/ immune cells in gingivitis are correct?**

A Plasma cells produce cytokines

B Macrophages produce antibodies

C Macrophages present antigen to lymphocytes

D Macrophages remove damaged tissue

E Polymorphonuclear cells (PMNs) secrete cytokines

10.45 **Which of the following clinical conditions predispose patients with impaired/defective neutrophil function to severe periodontitis?**

A Diabetes mellitus

B Papillon–Lefèvre syndrome

C Ehlers Danlos syndrome

D Chédiak–Higashi syndrome

E Hypophosphatasia

10.46 **Which of the following are appropriate scores and treatment according to the Basic Periodontal Examination (BPE)? The worst results per sextant are included as given below:**

A The coloured band on the probe is completely visible but there is bleeding on probing on a lower right first permanent molar – this would give a score of 3

B The coloured area totally disappears on probing on an upper left second permanent molar – this would give a score of 4

C An overhang on the margin of a restoration on a lower left first permanent molar would give a score of 2

D On probing an upper right central incisor, the pocket (the coloured area on the probe) partially disappears – this would give a score of 3

E The appropriate treatment for BPE score of 3 is oral hygiene instruction (OHI), scaling and root planing

10.44 CDE

Plasma cells produce antibodies and macrophages produce cytokines. PMNs secrete cytokines and inflammatory mediators. They also kill bacteria by intra-cellular and extra-cellular methods.

10.45 ABD

Ehlers Danlos syndrome and hypophosphatasia are associated with abnormal collagen formation, which then leads to periodontal destruction.

10.46 BCDE

The probe used is a World Health Organization (WHO) periodontal probe with a ball end with a diameter of 0.5 mm and a coloured band 3.5–5.5 mm from the tip. The scoring system is shown in the table.

Score	Disease	Treatment
0	No disease	
1	Gingival bleeding, no overhangs or calculus, pockets < 3.5 mm	OHI
2	No pockets > 3.5 mm, subgingival calculus present or subgingival overhangs	OHI, scaling and correction of any iatrogenic factors
3	Pockets within colour-coded area, ie > 3.5 – < 5.5 mm	OHI, scaling and root planing
4	Colour-coded area disappears, pockets > 5.5 mm	OHI, scaling, root planing with or without surgery

10.47 Necrotising gingivitis (necrotising ulcerative gingivitis or NUG):

A   Most commonly affects the first molars

B   Is characterised by interproximal necrosis (tips of papillae)

C   Is commoner in males

D   Is a Gram-positive anaerobic infection

E   Usually produces a characteristic odour

10.48 Management of a patient with NUG may include:

A   20% chlorhexidine mouthwashes twice daily

B   Hydrogen peroxide mouthwash

C   Vigorous toothbrushing

D   Metronidazole 200–400 mg three times daily for 5 days

E   Triamcinolone acetonide (Adcortyl) in Orabase gel applied topically to the lesions

10.49 Which of the following features would suggest that an abscess on a single-rooted tooth was periodontal rather than pulpal in origin?

A   The tooth in question is non-vital

B   The tooth in question is vital

C   There is pain on lateral movement of the tooth

D   There is pain on vertical movement of the tooth

E   There is loss of the alveolar crest height on the radiograph

10.47 BE

Necrotising ulcerative gingivitis most commonly affects the mandibular incisor region and unerupted third molars. There is no predilection for either sex. NUG is a Gram-negative anaerobic infection, and there is usually a foetor-ex-ore, although this is not pathognomic of NUG as it can occur in other pathological conditions of the oral cavity.

10.48 BD

Management of NUG includes removing soft and mineralised deposits in the mouth and improving oral hygiene. However, the lesions are often very painful so patients are not able to use a toothbrush in the initial period. Thus chemical debridement is often used. Mouthwashes such as 0.2% chlorhexidine or hydrogen peroxide are used, as is metronidazole systemically. Triamcinolone acetonide (Adcortyl) in Orobase is a steroid-based preparation that is not indicated for NUG lesions.

10.49 BCE

An abscess originating from the pulp is usually associated with a non-vital tooth, and the tooth is painful on vertical movements. With periodontal abscesses the tooth may be vital and the tooth is painful on lateral movements, and there is often loss of alveolar bone height on radiographs.

10.50 When assessing tooth mobility:

A   Movement of a crown of a tooth in the horizontal plane of less than 0.2 mm is considered normal

B   Grade 1 means movement of the crown of a tooth in the horizontal plane is 0.2–1 mm

C   Grade 2 means movement of the crown of a tooth in the horizontal plane is greater than 1 mm

D   Grade 3 means movement of the crown of a tooth in the horizontal plane is greater than 3 mm

E   Grade 3 means movement of the crown of a tooth in the vertical plane

10.51 Which of the following factors may have a bearing on the measurements recorded on probing pocket depths?

A   The degree of force applied to the probe

B   The thickness of the probe

C   The degree of inflammatory exudate in the gingival soft tissues

D   The bacterial flora in the pocket

E   The amount of gingival crevicular fluid produced

10.52 Regarding dental calculus:

A   It is mineralised dental plaque

B   It is a primary cause of periodontitis

C   The outer surface remains covered by a layer of plaque

D   It is composed of hydroxyapatite

E   It forms when plaque is mineralized from calcium and carbonate ions in the saliva

10.50 ABCE

Tooth mobility is often classified in the following manner:

- Grade 1 – movement of the crown of a tooth in the horizontal plane 0.2–1 mm
- Grade 2 – movement of the crown of a tooth in the horizontal plane greater than 1 mm
- Grade 3 – movement of the crown of a tooth in the vertical plane

10.51 ABC

Periodontal pocket depth probing can be inconsistent due to a number of reasons including: the thickness of the probe; the amount of pressure applied; the angulation of the probe in the pocket; the (mal)position of the probe; and the amount of inflammatory exudate in the soft tissues. The amount of crevicular fluid and the bacterial flora in the pocket do not influence measurement of pocket depths.

10.52 ACD

The primary cause of periodontitis is plaque not calculus. It forms when plaque is mineralised by calcium and phosphate ions in the saliva.

10.53 A patient attends your practice wearing dentures with a reduced vertical dimension. What complaints may they have due to the reduced vertical dimension?

   A Difficulty with 'S' sounds

   B Poor appearance showing too little teeth

   C Clicking of teeth when talking

   D Sunken lower face, elderly looking appearance

   E Ill defined pain on the lower denture bearing area that settles when the dentures are removed

10.54 Which of the following are important to assess before planning treatment that involves an implant-retained lower denture?

   A History of alcohol intake

   B Oral hygiene

   C Quality of bone

   D Position of maxillary sinus

   E Past history of mouth cancer

10.55 Which of the following are indications for copy dentures?

   A To make a spare set of dentures

   B There is a loss of retention, but the rest of the features of the dentures are acceptable

   C Excessive wear of the occlusal surfaces

   D Where the patient lisps

   E Inadequate lip support

10.53 BD

Patients with reduced freeway space often complain of an aged appearance and not showing enough teeth. They may get tired with chewing due to increased masticatory effort being needed. S sounds are not affected by the change in vertical dimension. People wearing dentures with increased vertical dimension often complain of points A, C and E. They may also say that they are 'Showing too much teeth' or their 'Mouth is full of teeth'.

10.54 BCE

A moderate intake of alcohol is not a contraindication for implants but a history of smoking is – as it affects the rate of success of implants. The oral hygiene status and the quality of bone should both be assessed prior to treatment planning. A previous history of mouth cancer is important, in particular, if the patient has received radiotherapy with the risk of osteoradionecrosis. The position of the maxillary sinus is irrelevant.

10.55 ABC

Copy dentures are used to reproduce the favourable aspects of a set of dentures while improving certain features such as occlusion. They are used when patients have had good denture wearing experience with that particular denture. Hence if a patient lisps or there is inadequate lip support some alteration of the polished surfaces of the new dentures would be required.

10.56 Over-dentures:

   A Are contra-indicated in patients with cleft palates

   B Are contra-indicated in patients with inadequate inter-arch space

   C May be indicated when converting a partially dentate patient to a complete denture wearer

   D Are indicated in patients with uncontrolled periodontal disease

   E May be indicated in patients with attrition

10.57 Regarding Kennedy classification for partially edentulous arches:

   A A patient with upper right 8765 and upper left 34567 would be a described as Kennedy Class 4

   B A patient with lower right 54321 and lower left 1234 would be described as Kennedy Class 4

   C A patient with a lower right 76 321 and lower left 123 567 would be described as Kennedy Class 2

   D A patient with a lower right 76 321 and lower left 123 567 would be described as Kennedy Class 3 modification 1

   E A patient with a lower right 87654321 and lower left 123 would be described as a Kennedy Class 3

10.58 Supposed advantages of over-dentures over complete dentures include:

   A Better aesthetics

   B Preservation of alveolar bone

   C The patient will have greater sensory feedback

   D Increased biting forces

   E More reproducible retruded jaw relations

10.56 BCE

Over-dentures are contra-indicated in patients with poor oral hygiene, uncontrolled caries or periodontal disease. There is no reason why a patient with a cleft palate should not have an over-denture and they may be a useful treatment option.

10.57 AD

The Kennedy classification is used to describe partially dentate arches:

- Class 1 – bilateral free end saddles
- Class 2 – one free end saddle
- Class 3 – a unilateral bounded saddle
- Class 4 – a single bounded saddle anterior to the abutment teeth

The classification is based on the most posterior edentulous area, but third molars are not included. A modification, (additional edentulous area), can be added to classes 1–3 when there are other missing teeth. Hence a patient with lower right 54321 and lower left 1234 would be described as Kennedy class 1, a patient with a lower right 87654321 and lower left 123 would be described as a Kennedy class 2.

10.58 BCDE

The aesthetics of complete dentures and over-dentures are comparable. As teeth are retained the patient has greater sensory feedback than when wearing complete dentures. Proprioception is believed to be enhanced and hence there is improved ability to reproduce retruded jaw relations with probable increased chewing thresholds.

10.59 The advantages of immediate dentures are:

A   The existing occlusion can be used for jaw registration purposes

B   The person does not have to be seen without teeth

C   They may act as a haemostatic aid following extractions

D   They usually work out cheaper for the patient

E   They slow down alveolar bone resorption

10.60 Which of the following are potential problems in patients with edentulous maxillae and only lower anterior teeth?

A   Flabby or fibrous upper ridge

B   Anterior seal of upper denture

C   Differential support and retention required in upper denture

D   Lower anterior teeth often worn down because of inadequate vertical height

E   Stability of upper denture

10.61 Surveying of casts for denture design:

A   Is carried out for complete and partial dentures

B   Is only carried out for cobalt-chrome dentures

C   Is used to determine the occlusal vertical dimension

D   Is used to determine undercuts with respect to the path of insertion of a denture

E   Is carried out with the model at right angles to the analyser rod

10.59 ABC

Immediate dentures do have the big psychological advantage that the person does not have to go around without teeth. However, because changes occur in the hard and soft tissues following extraction of teeth the dentures will need adjustment to retain their comfort and fit. This often ends up being more costly as relines need to be carried out or new dentures made. Placing dentures over the alveolar ridges does not reduce bone resorption.

10.60 ACE

Posterior seal of the upper denture is often a problem, as the lower anterior teeth cause the upper denture to tip. There is often over-eruption of the lower anterior teeth causing problems with occlusal plane. The greater force exerted by the natural teeth may lead to flabby ridge formation.

10.61 D

Surveying is carried out to determine undercuts and guide planes and find a path of insertion for a partial denture. It is not used for complete dentures but is carried out for all partial dentures irrespective of construction material.

10.62 Regarding the occlusion of complete dentures:

A   It is desirable to create dentures with canine guidance

B   It is desirable to create dentures with group function

C   It is desirable to create dentures with balanced articulation

D   It is desirable to create dentures with balanced occlusion

E   The occlusion should try to re-create what the patient had naturally

10.63 Regarding partial denture clasps:

A   In order to be functional they must be resisted by a non-retentive clasp arm/component

B   Cast cobalt-chrome clasps need to engage undercuts of greater than 0.25 mm

C   Wrought gold clasps are less flexible than stainless steel clasps

D   The shorter the clasp the more flexible it will be

E   Gingivally approaching clasps are less conspicuous than occlusally approaching clasps

10.64 Regarding connectors in partial dentures:

A   They hold the various parts of the denture together

B   They do not contribute to retention or support of the denture

C   Lingual bars are only used when there is less than 7 mm of space between the floor of the mouth and the gingival margin

D   A sublingual bar is more rigid than a lingual bar

E   Lingual bars are contra-indicated if the lower incisors are proclined

10.62 CD

When constructing complete dentures it is desirable to create both balanced occlusion and balanced articulation. Balanced occlusion means bilateral even contact between the upper and lower dentures in the intercuspal position and balanced articulation means bilateral even contact between the upper and lower dentures in lateral and protrusive movements. This helps maintain the stability of the dentures.

Canine guidance and group function describe the posterior occlusion of the working side teeth during lateral excursions in dentate people. Canine guidance will cause a denture to tip and is not desirable, group function is slightly better, but the ideal is balanced articulation. The patient's natural occlusion is not reproduced in dentures.

10.63 AE

Cast cobalt-chrome clasps need to engage undercuts of less than 0.25 mm as they are stiff and liable to fracture. Wrought gold clasps are more flexible than stainless steel and cast cobalt-chrome clasps, and the longer a clasp is the more flexible it will be.

10.64 AD

Connectors can contribute to support and retention. Lingual bars are only used when there is more than 7 mm of space between the floor of the mouth and the gingival margin, as they need 3 mm clearance from the gingival margin. Lingual bars are contra-indicated if the lower incisors are retroclined.

Index

Notes